Baillière's

# CLINICAL ANAESTHESIOLOGY

INTERNATIONAL PRACTICE AND RESEARCH

Baillière's

# CLINICAL ANAESTHESIOLOGY

INTERNATIONAL PRACTICE AND RESEARCH

Volume 12/Number 3
September 1998

# Pre-anaesthetic Care

W. F. LIST MD
H. METZLER MD
*Guest Editors*

Baillière Tindall
**London Philadelphia Sydney Tokyo Toronto**

This book is printed on acid-free paper.

Baillière Tindall Harcourt Brace Publishers International
24–28 Oval Road
London NW1 7DX, UK

Harcourt Brace & Company
The Curtis Center, Independence Square West,
Philadelphia, PA 19106–3399, USA

Harcourt Brace & Company
55 Horner Avenue
Toronto, Ontario M8Z 4X6, Canada

Harcourt Brace & Company Australia
30–52 Smidmore Street, Marrickville, NSW 2204, Australia

Harcourt Brace & Company Japan Inc
Ichibancho Central Building,
22–1 Ichibancho, Chiyoda-ku, Tokyo 102, Japan



ISSN 0950–3501

ISBN 0–7020–2536–4 (single copy)



*Baillière's Clinical Anaesthesiology* is published four times each year by Baillière Tindall.
Prices for Volume 12 (1998) are:

| TERRITORY | ANNUAL SUBSCRIPTION | SINGLE ISSUE |
|---|---|---|
| Europe including UK | £105.00 (Institutional) post free<br>£85.00 (Individual) post free | £31.00 post free |
| All other countries | Consult your local Harcourt Brace & Company office | |

Managing Editor: Seán Duggan
Production Editor: Garry Griffin
Assistant Editor: Chris Hammond
Journals Publisher: Martin Delahunty

Editorial office: Baillière Tindall, c/o Harcourt Brace & Company, 24–28 Oval Road, London NW1 7DX, UK. Email: journals@harcourtbrace.com

*Baillière's Clinical Anaesthesiology* is covered in Index Medicus, Current Contents/Clinical Medicine, Current Contents/Life Sciences, the Science Citation Index, SciSearch, Research Alert and EMBASE/Excerpta Medica.

*Baillière's Clinical Anaesthesiology* was published from 1972 to 1986 as *Clinics in Anaesthesiology*

Typeset by Phoenix Photosetting, Chatham. Printed and bound in Great Britain by the University Printing House, Cambridge, UK.

# Contributors to this issue

**PIERRE CORIAT** MD, FANZCA, Professor and Chairman, Groupe Hospitalier Pitié-Salpêtrière, 47–83 Boulevard de l'Hôpital, 75651 Paris Cedex 13, France.

**WOLFGANG F. DICK** FRCA, Director, International Trauma Anaesthesia Critical Care Society; Vice-chairman, European Resuscitation Council; Hon. Secretary, World Association of Disaster and Emergency Medicine; President, German Association of Critical Care Medicine (DIVI); Chairman, Department of Anaesthesiology, Klinik für Anästhesiologie, Klinikum der Universität Mainz, Langenbeckstr. 1, 55131 Mainz, Germany.

**ROBERT O. FENECK** MB, BS, FRCA, Consultant Anaesthesiologist and Hon. Senior Lecturer, St. Thomas's Hospital, Lambeth Palace Road, London SE1 7EH, UK.

**LEE A. FLEISHER** MD, Associate Professor of Anesthesiology and Critical Care Medicine, Joint Appointment in Medicine (Cardiology) and Health Policy and Management, Johns Hopkins Medical Institutions, Carnegie 442, 600 North Wolfe Street, Baltimore, Maryland 21287, USA.

**SUSANNE E. GASSMAYR** MD, Resident, Department of Anaesthesiology and Intensive Care Medicine, Karl-Franzens-University Graz, Auenbruggerplatz 29, A-8036 Graz, Austria.

**GORDON L. GIBBY** MD, Associate Professor of Anesthesiology and Medicine, University of Florida College of Medicine, Department of Anesthesiology, PO Box 100254, Gainesville, FL 32610-0254, USA.

**HANS GOMBOTZ** MD, Associate Professor, Department of Anaesthesiology and Intensive Care Medicine, University of Graz, Auenbruggerplatz 29, A-8036 Graz, Austria.

**LOUISE GOUILLE** MD, Staff Anaesthesiologist, Groupe Hospitalier Pitié-Salpêtrière, 47–83 Boulevard de l'Hôpital, 75651 Paris Cedex 13, France.

**NIKOLAUS GRAVENSTEIN** MD, The Jerome H. Medell, MD, Professor and Chairman of Anesthesiology, University of Florida College of Medicine, Department of Anesthesiology, PO Box 100254, Gainesville, FL 32610-0254, USA.

**WOLFGANG KRÖLL** MD, PhD, Associate Professor, Department of Anaesthesiology and Intensive Care Medicine, Karl-Franzens-University Graz, Auenbruggerplatz 29, A-8036 Graz, Austria.

**PATRICIA LEUFKE** Assistant, Institut für Anaesthesiologie und operative Intensivmedizin, Klinikum Stadt Hanau, Leimenstr. 20, 63450 Hanau, Germany.

**WERNER F. LIST** MD, Professor and Chairman, Department of Anaesthesiology and Intensive Care Medicine, University of Graz, Auenbruggerplatz 29, A-8036 Graz, Austria.

**HELFRIED METZLER** MD, Professor of Anaesthesiology, Department of Anaesthesiology and Intensive Care Medicine, University of Graz, Auenbruggerplatz 29, A-8036 Graz, Austria.

**PETER M. OSSWALD** MD, Director, Institut für Anaesthesiologie und operative Intensivmedizin, Klinikum Stadt Hanau, Leimenstr. 20, 63450 Hanau, Germany.

**THOMAS PASCH** MD, Professor and Chairman, Institute of Anaesthesiology, University Hospital Zürich, Rämistrasse 100, CH-8091 Zürich, Switzerland.

**GERHARD PRAUSE** MD, Associate Professor of Anaesthesiology and Intensive Care Medicine, Department of Anaesthesiology and Intensive Care Medicine, University of Graz, Auenbruggerplatz 29, A-8036 Graz, Austria.

**OLAV SWARS** MD, Assistant resident, Institut für Anaesthesiologie und operative Intensivmedizin, Klinikum Stadt Hanau, Leimenstr. 20, 63450 Hanau, Germany.

**ANDREAS ZOLLINGER** MD, Consultant and Senior Lecturer, Institute of Anaesthesiology, University Hospital Zürich, Rämistrasse 100, CH-8091 Zürich, Switzerland.

# Table of contents

## PREVIOUS ISSUES

Vol. 10, No. 2 1996
**Quality Assurance and Risk Management in Anaesthesia**
A. R. Aitkenhead

Vol. 10, No. 3 1996
**Neuroprotection**
J. A. Stamford & L. Strunin

Vol. 10, No. 4 1996
**Paediatric Anaesthesia**
S. G. E. Lindahl

Vol. 11, No. 1 1997
**Plasma Volume Support**
H. Haljamäe

Vol. 11, No. 2 1997
**Blood, Blood Products and Blood Saving Techniques**
V. Kretschmer & B. Blauhut

Vol. 11, No. 3 1997
**Burns**
J. Kinsella

Vol. 11, No. 4 1997
**Arterial Hypertension**
K. Skarvan

Vol. 12, No. 1 1998
**Chronic Pain Relief**
M. Zenz

Vol. 12, No. 2 1998
**Drug Interactions**
J. G. Bovill

## FORTHCOMING ISSUE

Vol. 12, No. 4 1998
**Transoesophageal Echocardiography**
J. Poelaert

# Preface

The anaesthesiologist cannot delegate his or her right and duty of evaluating a surgical patient pre-operatively. Only the anaesthesiologist has the special knowledge about the pharmacology of anaesthetic agents and anaesthesia techniques to assess the specific medical problems in relation to anaesthesia and surgery. An expert evaluation of the surgical patient is needed as to his or her acute or chronic diseases in addition to the surgical lesion. The physical status of the patient and the anaesthesia risk also then have to be evaluated according to an accepted scoring system.

The current risk of a patient for an anaesthesia-induced death is according to newer statistics 1 : 185 000 for in hospital patients (Lunn and Devlin, 1987, *Lancet*). Statistics in patients with anaesthesia in ambulant surgery show an even lower anaesthesia mortality. The type of surgery, pre-existing disease and anaesthesia are determining factors of outcome; the patient's health status is the most important of these.

In a study on Finnish patients Tikkanen and Hovi Viander (1995, *Acta Anaesthesiologica Scandinavica*) found that internal disease in surgical patients was more than 20 times more often the reason for post-operative mortality than anaesthesia or surgery. Our own experiences with more than 100 000 pre-operative surgical patients have shown that about 40% of our patients have severe medical disease in addition to their surgical problem. About 8% of these patients can be improved as to their medical status before going to anaesthesia (Prause et al, 1998, *Acta Anaesthesiologica Scandinavica*).

It is the duty of an anaesthesia department to organize an efficient pre-operative patient evaluation. Depending on the size of the department different forms, for example bed-side interview, consulting hour or pre-operative evaluation clinic, have been proven successful. The first suggestion for a pre-operative anaesthesia clinic came from Lee (1949, *Anaesthesia*). It is this form of patient evaluation that is most promising and effective for a larger anaesthesia institutions.

This book on pre-anaesthetic care contains an overview of different approaches in Europe, for example standard screening or minimal screening sets, and transatlantic differences in views on pre-operative evaluation. An epidemiological study of anaesthesia relevant electrocardiogram (ECG) changes in different patient groups and healthy firemen should influence the long-standing discussion on routine screening, cut-off age or demand ECG evaluation towards routine ECG pre-operative screening. It has to be stressed that there are only few prospective studies about screening and outcome and that most positions held and standards set are not based on studies but possibly on economic considerations. Cost containment is of increasing importance in the practice of anaesthesia. The need for further prospective studies of pre-operative patient evaluation and outcome has to be stressed.

After this introduction to pre-anaesthetic care, the evaluation of special high-risk patients is described. Separate chapters deal with cardiac risk patients for non-cardiac surgery and possible pre-operative cardiac interventions as well as the patient under chronic medication. New ideas and experiences about pulmonary risk patients and their care are dealt with in contrast to previously held beliefs. The pre-anaesthetic care of the emergency patient is also a frequent concern but rarely discussed.

Scoring and outcome, as well as the pre-operative optimization of haemoglobin and the critical haematocrit are addressed within further chapters.

Finally, new guidelines on pre-anaesthetic fasting, pre-medication and the documentation of pre-anaesthetic findings should complete the extensive information on pre-anaesthetic care of surgical patients.

W.F.LIST
H. METZLER

## REFERENCES

Lee A (1949) The anaesthetic outpatient clinic. *Anaesthesia* **4:** 169.

Lunn JN & Devlin MB (1987) Lessons from the confidential enquiry into perioperative deaths in three NHS regions. *Lancet* **2:** 1384–1386.

Prause G, Ratzenhofer-Komenda B, Smolle-Juettner F et al (1998) Operations on patients deemed 'unfit for operation and anaesthesia': what are the consequences? *Acta Anaesthesiologica Scandinavica* **42:** 316–322.

Tikkanen J & Hovi-Viander M (1995) Death associated with anaesthesia and surgery in Finland in 1986 compared to 1975. *Acta Anaesthesiologica Scandinavica* **38:** 262–267.

# 1

# The pre-operative clinic

WERNER F. LIST MD
Professor and Chairman

GERHARD PRAUSE MD
Associate Professor of Anaesthesiology and Intensive Care Medicine
*Department of Anaesthesiology and Intensive Care Medicine, University of Graz, Auenbruggerplatz 29, A-8036 Graz, Austria*

The pre-operative examination is an indisputable duty of the anaesthesiologist. It can be performed in three different ways: the bed-side visit, the anaesthesiological consulting hour and the pre-operative clinic. The bed-side visit enables the anaesthesiologist scheduled for giving anaesthesia to introduce himself or herself to the patient. There is no additional cost for staff and equipment; however, the investigation is limited to a cursory interpretation of previous investigations and examinations. The best way to perform a pre-operative anaesthesiological examination is the pre-operative clinic. The staff of the pre-operative clinic comprises an anaesthesist, a nurse and a secretary. The examination is standardized and therefore easy to perform, easy to teach and easy to control. It includes an interview with the patient, a physical examination and the evaluation of several screening tests, if available (laboratory tests, chest X-ray, lung function and resting electrocardiogram). The complete examination enables the decision on whether the patient is fit for anaesthesia or not to be made. In a patient declared to be unfit the pre-operative condition has to be optimized and additional tests or consultants are required to rule out severe pre-operative diseases suspected on the basis of the pre-operative anaesthesiological investigation. If the suspicion is not confirmed, the patient proceeds to operation. If concomitant diseases are verified the surgical intervention is postponed until the patient's condition has been optimized. The costs of the pre-operative clinic are higher, mainly because of the need for additional anaesthesiological staff. However, as the pre-operative clinic enables a thorough and complete evaluation in most cases, it is the optimal presentation of the discipline anaesthesia. In our experience it plays a major role in quality management of patient care.

**Key words:** pre-operative evaluation; organization; structure.

## STRUCTURE

A patient scheduled for surgery and anaesthesia has to be evaluated by an anaesthesiologist pre-operatively (Roizen, 1986; Downing and Tinker,

*Baillière's Clinical Anaesthesiology—*
Vol. 12, No. 3, September 1998
ISBN 0–7020–2536–4
0950–3501/98/030333 + 07 $12.00/00

1987; Opderbecke and Weißauer, 1987; Ahnefeld, 1997). This evaluation will include an interview and the evaluation of pre-existing findings from the patient's record as well as a physical examination. Theoretically, these requirements can be met by a number of different structures:

1. the bed-side visit,
2. the anaesthesiological consulting hour, and
3. the pre-operative anaesthesiological clinic.

During a pre-operative visit the anaesthesiologist has to introduce him- or herself to the patient, already scheduled for surgery on the following day (Peter and Lutz, 1973; Van Aken and Rolf, 1997). As a rule this consultation will be a bed-side talk on the ward, performed by the anaesthesiologist who is scheduled to give anaesthesia to the patient the following day. By establishing a personal contact between patient and anaesthesiologist this consultation will reduce the patient's anxiety. In some instances the investigation will be reduced to an interview focusing on data from the history and on current complaints. A thorough physical examination is not usually carried out; rather, reliance is placed on the findings from other specialists and on the cumulative data from the patient's record. Finally, a definitive decision about the patient's fitness and type of anaesthesia is made.

The personal relationship of the anaesthesiologist giving anaesthesia to the patient is mandatory and cannot be replaced by another pre-anaesthesia assessment. It does not require additional staff or additional technical equipment.

The anaesthesiological consulting hour enables the anaesthesiologist to evaluate pre-existing findings from the patient's record whereas the patients may ask questions about the anaesthesiologic management, complications and the peri-operative treatment (Nightingale and Lack, 1992; Ahnefeld, 1997). A consultation room is necessary, where investigations, for example spirometry, of electrocardiograms (ECGs) or others can be done. The anaesthesiologist present during the consulting hour may be the one actually giving anaesthesia to the patient; then the anaesthesiological consulting hour can replace the pre-operative bed-side visit.

Indisputably the best method of pre-anaesthesia care is a well-organized pre-operative anaesthesiological assessment unit or pre-anaesthesia clinic (Dick et al, 1978; List, 1982, 1990, 1992; Janecskó et al, 1983; List et al, 1985; Prause, 1994; Dick, 1997). Similarly to other specialists, the anaesthesiologist presents him- or herself as a member of a well-organized institution for peri-operative care. Ideally, the staff of the pre-operative assessment unit comprises an anaesthesiologist, a nurse and a secretary. Accordingly, the costs especially for the staff are high. Patients are evaluated according to their age with a fixed screening schedule, the pre-operative findings being documented on a special form. Investigations essential for the anaesthesiological assessment are performed at the unit to be used and only in case of special questions, for example cardiological or endocrinological, can the opinion of external consultants be sought. As a rule the examining physician is not the one who gives anaesthesia to these patients. The examination procedure has to be documented and can be easily communicated to residents and is well controllable, guaranteeing an optimal first step of the peri-operative quality assessment.

The patient's information about the peri-operative anaesthesiological management should be provided during the bed-side visit or consulting hour by the person giving anaesthesia. This is the best way, because anaesthesia-related problems and complications depend also on the choice of anaesthesia, a decision which can only be made by the anaesthesiologist.

The three pre-operative organizations are compared in Table 1.

**Table 1.** Comparison of the three pre-operative organizations.

| | Bed-side visit | Consulting hour | Pre-operative anaesthesiological clinic |
|---|---|---|---|
| Personnel | Physician | Physician | Physician, nurse and secretary |
| Equipment | None | Room and desk | Investigation room; room enabling the patient to dress and undress; desk; equipment (ECG apparatus, spirometer, blood gas check analyser, etc.) |
| Advantage | Personal contact | Personal contact, explanation and information, more time | Well-trained physician, systemic examination, good representation of anaesthesia |
| Disadvantage | Little time for physical examination | Only useful in small hospitals, can replace bed-side visit | Additional staff members, examiner will not give anaesthesia, bed-side visit necessary |
| Costs | None | Low | High |

## ORGANIZATION OF A PRE-OPERATIVE ANAESTHESIOLOGICAL ASSESSMENT UNIT

The pre-anaesthesia clinic is an important component of peri-operative care in an anaesthesiological department. As everyday routine usually confines anaesthesiologists to the operating theatres or intensive care unit, an institution allowing a direct contact with the patient for the purpose of anaesthesia is vital for patients as well as for physicians from other disciplines.

A rapid turnover of pre-operative patients in a big institution is only possible with an adequate organization of the unit. The room should be divided into a waiting zone, a cabin enabling the patient to dress and undress and the actual examination area. The latter must be dimensioned in a way that also enables the examination of bed-ridden patients in their beds.

As most of the investigations required for pre-anaesthesiological assessment will be done in the same unit, ECG and spirometry equipment and a blood gas analyser as well as facilities enabling blood samples to be drawn are necessary. Close proximity to a biochemical laboratory is useful. Both physician and the secretary need a desk, to evaluate the patient's record and for computerized documentation of the findings, respectively.

The course of a typical pre-operative anaesthesiological assessment at the Department of Anaesthesiology and Intensive Care Medicine in Graz would be as follows.

## Data acquisition, screening tests and evaluation of record

After the patient's personal data have been taken by the secretary, electrocardiography, a simple lung function test and, if necessary, blood gas analysis are done by the nurse. In the case of pathological findings in the resting ECG, additional tests can be performed (e.g. prolonged ECG recording, inspiratory ECG evaluating signs of a post-infarctial scar) (List, 1990). As a screening for the patient's lung function, a short spirometry is sufficient. Meanwhile, the physician studies the patient's record, evaluating the impact of pre-existing findings on the fitness for anaesthesia for the planned type of operation.

## Interview

The patient's interview focuses on previous operations and peri-operative complications, medication, personal tolerance of previous anaesthesia and irregularities of anaesthesia tolerance in relatives. Special attention is paid to a history of peri-operative thromboembolic events and to the proneness to allergic reactions. The further interview is mainly directed at cardiac problems, i.e. a history of myocardial infarction or 'heart attacks', evaluating heart pain while at rest or during exercise or cardiac syncopes (Eagle et al, 1996). In the case of previous myocardial infarction the documentation of the interval since the event is essential (Goldman et al, 1977; Goldman, 1995).

The patient's exercise capacity is a subjective estimation; the physician grades this description into four classes according to the exercise index of the New York Heart Association for cardiac patients (New York Heart Association, 1985). Finally the patient is asked about severe dysfunctions or about those of other organs, especially of lungs, kidneys and liver, about metabolic disorders, symptoms of arterial hypoperfusion, and about his or her personal habits, especially concerning smoking and drinking.

The structure of the interview is summarized in Table 2.

## Physical examination

The estimation of the general condition is subjective, being dependent on the experience of the examiner. Exploration of the dental status is done and any information for the patient about possible problems following

**Table 2.** Structure of the pre-operative interview.

| |
|---|
| Previous operations |
| Previous peri-operative complications |
| Known anaesthetic irregularities |
| Cardiac disturbances |
| Previous myocardial infarction |
| Myocardial infarction within the last 6 months |
| Arterial hypertension |
| Syncopes |
| Proneness to thrombembolism |
| History of stroke |
| Arteriosclerosis |
| Diabetes mellitus |
| Kidney disease |
| Smoking and drinking habits |
| Allergic disposition |
| Dental situation |

intubation is given in order to rule out legal action in case of iatrogenic damage. The auscultation of heart and lungs is mandatory and done in each case. Attention is paid to liver size, oedema of the lower extremities and distension of the cervical veins as indirect signs of cardiac dysfunction.

## Final evaluation

On the basis of the findings from the patient's history, from screening tests, from the records and from the physical examination and keeping in mind the notes taken during the interview, the physician decides whether the patient is fit for anaesthesia and operation. In the case of pathological findings such as mild pulmonary obstruction or varicose veins, an amendment of the current therapy or additional investigations, respectively, are suggested, although the patient is declared 'fit for anaesthesia and for operation'.

If severe disturbances are suspected or documented, however, further exploration and/or therapy is requested and the patient is declared to be 'primarily unfit for anaesthesia and operation' (Downing and Tinker, 1987; Prause et al, 1998). In this case the operation has to be postponed until the necessary investigations and tests have been performed and/or until therapy has been initiated. A second evaluation of these patients is necessary.

All relevant data for anaesthesia are recorded on the pre-operative assessment protocol (Prause et al, 1990; Prause, 1994).

A final statement describes the essential findings and the patient's anaesthetic assessment, classified according to the American Society of Anesthesiology (ASA) physical status (Meyer, 1941; Dripps, 1963). The cardiac risk index (CRI) of Goldman is calculated automatically by the computer system and is also documented. The mean duration of one examination is about 15 min (range: 5–30 min).

The pre-operative assessment is ended with an informative talk about the procedures necessary before, during and after anaesthesia, giving the patient the chance to ask questions and thus to reduce his or her apprehension.

## SCREENING TEST OR ON DEMAND?

Many authors disapprove of routine pre-operative tests and demand tests only in selected patients (Lutz et al, 1983; Blery et al, 1986; Roizen, 1986; Tarnow, 1996). They argue that the low percentage of pathological findings in patients deemed 'healthy' by physical examination and interview does not justify the expense. These critics define the patient's threshold age (40 years and/or 60 years) and distinguish between male and female patients when deciding to perform screening tests. Although in principle younger patients are actually less likely to show pathological findings during routine tests, several problems arise when adopting a selective testing mode. The threshold of age itself gives rise to the question, 'is a patient aged 42 years much more endangered than a 39 year old patient?'. Furthermore, with two age-based thresholds and a difference according to gender six groups are created, each of which requires a different set of pre-operative tests. Finally, the necessity for additional tests and a possible time delay are likely in this setting. It will cause a frequent need for a second evaluation, thus delaying the operation and increasing expense.

A selected screening programme equal for all patients is easily performed and enables a ready availability for all tests. One representative test enables an evaluation of the vital organ function in about 94% of patients (Prause et al, 1990, 1998). The set of pre-operative routine screening tests includes the following:

- lung function (vital capacity, forced expiratory volume in 1 second)
- ECG

Laboratory tests include

- blood cell count (haemoglobin or haematocrit)
- electrolytes (potassium and sodium)
- kidney function (creatinine)
- blood glucose
- liver function (gamma-Glutamyl-transferase ($\gamma$GT))
- chest roentgenogram after 40 years

## REFERENCES

Ahnefeld FW (1997) Anästhesie—Optimale perioperative Betreuung? *Anaesthesist* **46 (supplement 2):** 571–574.

Van Aken H & Rolf N (1997) Preoperative evaluation and preparation—the anaesthesiologists' view. *Anaesthesist* **46 (supplement 2):** 580–584.

Blery Y, Chappak Y, Szatan M, et al (1986) Evaluation of a protocol for selective ordering of preoperative tests. *Lancet* **1:** 139–141.

Dick WF (1997) The preoperative anaesthesia clinic—a solution? *Anaesthesist* **46 (supplement 2):** 596–598.

Dick W, Ahnefeld FW, Fricke M et al (1978) Die Anaesthesieambulanz. Erfahrungen mit einer neuen Organisationsform der pränarkotischen Untersuchung und Beratung. *Anaesthesist* **27:** 450–458.

Downing JW & Tinker JH (1987) Fitness for anaesthesia: who decides? *Lancet* **1(8529):** 387 (letter).

Dripps RD (1963) New classification of physical status. *Anaesthesiology* **24:** 111.

Eagle KE, Brundage BH, Chaitman BR et al (1996) Guidelines for perioperative cardiovascular evaluation for non-cardiac surgery. *Journal of the American College of Cardiologists* **27(4):** 910–948.

Goldman L (1995) Cardiac risk in noncardiac surgery: an update. *Anesthesia and Analgesia* **80:** 810–820.

Goldman L, Caldera DL, Nussbaum SR et al (1977) Multifactorial index of cardiac risk in noncardiac surgical procedures. *New England Journal of Medicine* **297:** 845–850.

Janecskó M, Unk É & Pálos L (1983) Unsere Erfahrungen mit der Anaesthesieambulanz. *Anaesthesist* **32:** 174–176.

List WF (1982) The preoperative anaesthesia clinic. *Current Reviews in Clinical Anesthesia*, vol. 3. Miami, FL, USA.

List WF (1990) Organisationsformen der präoperativen Befunderhebung. *Anästhesiologie und Intensivmedizin* **31:** 307–309.

List WF (1992) Vorbereitung des Patienten. In Doenicke A, Kettler D, List WF et al (eds) *Anästhesiologie, Lehrbuch der Anästhesiologie und Intensivmedizin 1*, 6th edn, pp 8–35. Berlin: Springer.

List WF, Kröll W & Filzwieser G (1985) Perioperatives Risiko schwerkranker chirurgischer Patienten. *Anaesthesist* **34:** 612–618.

Lutz H, Osswald PM & Bender HJ (1983) Ist die Forderung nach einem präoperativen Routine-untersuchungsprogramm (RUP) gerechtfertigt? *Anästhesie Intensivtherapie Notfallmedizin* **18:** 153–155.

Meyer S (1941) Grading of patients for surgical procedures. *Anaesthesiology* **2:** 281–285.

New York Heart Association (1985) Nomenclature and criteria for diagnosis of diseases of the heart and blood vessels. *Datenbuch Anästhesiologie*, vol. 1, p. 390. In Nemes C, Niemer M, Noack G (eds). Stuttgart: Gustav Fischer Verlag.

Nightingale JJ & Lack JA (1992) The preoperative anaesthetic visit. *Anaesthesia* **47:** 801–802.

Opderbecke HW & Weiβauer W (1987) Die Pflicht des Anästhesisten zur Voruntersuchung und die Fachgebietsgrenzen. Eine Urteilssprechung. *Anästhesiologie und Intensivmedizin* **28:** 382–384.

Peter K & Lutz H (1973) Präoperative Befunderhebung. *Langenbeck Archiv fur Chirurgie* **334:** 681–687.

Prause G (1994) The preoperative outpatient clinic in Graz: the first 15 years. *Anaesthesist* **43:** 223–228.

Prause G, Gombotz H, Rehak P & List WF (1990) The preoperative clinic—a probable use for a personal computer. *Anaesthesist* **39:** 186–190.

Prause G, Ratzenhofer-Komenda B, Krenn H, et al (1998) Operations on patients deemed 'Unfit for operation and anaesthesia': what are the consequences? *Acta Anaesthesiologica Scandinavica* **42:** 490–495.

Roizen MF (1986) Routine preoperative evaluation. In Miller RD (ed.) *Anaesthesia*, pp 225–253. New York: Churchill Livingstone.

Tarnow J (1996) Nutzen und Kosten präoperativer 'Screening'-Untersuchungen aus anästhesiologischer Sicht. *Anästhesiologie und Intensivmedizin* **37:** 268–272.

2

# Epidemiology of pathological electrocardiogram findings

WERNER F. LIST MD

Professor and Chairman

GERHARD PRAUSE MD

Associate Professor of Anaesthesiology and Intensive Care Medicine

*Department of Anaesthesiology and Intensive Care Medicine, University of Graz, Auenbruggerplatz 29, A-8036 Graz, Austria*

A 12-lead electrocardiogram (ECG) allows the recognition of cardiac diseases that may have evolved without causing subjective disturbances. ST changes, bundle branch blocks or left ventricular hypertrophy as well as arrhythmias or premature ectopies are the most important findings. In younger patients the detection of a pre-excitation syndrome (especially Wolff–Parkinson–White) is essential, as it does require special therapeutic management. At our pre-operative clinic a resting ECG is part of the screening programme. The data of 18 939 patients were evaluated over a 3 year period, divided into two categories, with (category I) or without (category II) previous cardiac disturbances in their history. In comparison the resting ECGs of 10 523 healthy firemen (category III) were evaluated. The percentage of pathological ECG findings in the patients scheduled for non-cardiac surgery was high. Depending on the decade of their life, 9.5–45.2% of subjects in category I (without any previous cardiac disturbances) and 13.2–80.2% in category II had a pathological ECG. In contrast, only 1.6–4.2% of subjects in category III had pathological ECG findings. The statement that the percentage of relevant pathological findings is increasing with age can be emphasized although a threshold cannot actually be defined: there is no difference in the incidence of changes in the age groups from 40 to 60 years. On the other hand, surgical patients without any cardiac history showed an incidence of pathological findings of 7.6%. The ECG is an inexpensive, easy-to-perform non-invasive procedure. In combination with an exact physical examination and a careful judgement of the impact of the findings on anaesthesia it allows a reliable pre-operative evaluation.

**Key words:** pre-operative evaluation; electrocardiogram; epidemiology.

A 12-lead electrocardiogram (ECG) is currently recommended for adult patients before various operations requiring general anaesthesia (Elston and Taylor, 1984; List, 1984; Moorman et al, 1985; Goldberger and O'Kinsky,


ISBN 0-7020-2536-4
0950-3501/98/030341 + 07 $12.00/00

1986; Eagle et al, 1996). Some anaesthesiologists (Seymour et al, 1983; Roizen, 1986) set a cut-off age (between 40 and 60 years) for the necessity of a pre-operative ECG because it has been documented that the incidence of abnormal findings in the ECG increases exponentially with age. The argument against the ECG screening is that, although it is non-invasive and relatively inexpensive, this investigation carries problems. Mainly, the high incidence of false-positive results without any organic equivalent may give rise to time-consuming and even invasive procedures in the search for actually non-existing cardiac diseases.

On the other hand, ECG changes can be the first clue to life-threatening metabolic disorders (hyperkalaemia or hypokalaemia) and/or major underlying heart disease or unrecognized myocardial infarction. Furthermore, the pre-operative ECG could become an important baseline investigation which may later be referred to in the case of peri-operative complications, such as arrhythmia or ST changes.

In an epidemiological study we tried to evaluate the incidence of pre-operative pathological findings of the resting ECG of patients scheduled for elective non-cardiac surgery with and without subjective cardiac disturbances. A group of healthy firemen served as non-surgical controls. All three groups were screened for anaesthesia-relevant ECG changes. These anaesthesia-relevant ECG changes were defined as follows (Goldberger and O'Kinsky, 1986):

- previous infarction in the history;
- no sinus rhythm;
- more than 5 premature ventricular contractions (PVC)/min;
- left ventricular hypertrophy;
- ST changes;
- bundle branch block;
- Wolff–Parkinson–White (WPW) syndrome.

Other ECG abnormalities such as atrioventricular (AV) blocks of different grades, sinus disturbances and tachycardias, not identified to cause peri-operative problems, were disregarded in our epidemiological study. We tried to answer two questions.

1. Is there actually an age threshold for the occurrence of pathological ECG findings?
2. How many pathological changes are found in individuals without any subjective cardiac complaints?

## DATA ACQUISITION

A resting ECG is routinely obtained as a part of the standard evaluation for elective non-cardiac surgery in our pre-operative assessment unit (List, 1984; Prause, 1994). The findings were evaluated by an anaesthesiologist with additional qualification as general practitioner, which in Austria includes 12 months training in internal medicine. Pathological ECG findings were re-evaluated by a cardiologist in order to confirm the diagnosis by a second opinion. All data were stored automatically by a computer system (dBaseIII+) (Prause et al, 1990).

The standard evaluation programme assessing the fitness of firemen includes a resting ECG as well. The investigation was performed by a group of cardiologists. The data were stored in a computer system (UNIX).

The almost 30 000 subjects were grouped into three categories (surgical patients with and without cardiac history and healthy controls), and subdivided into five age groups, the corresponding percentages of pathological anaesthesia ECG findings being compared.

## RESULTS

During the observation period (1994–1996) 18 939 patients were evaluated at our pre-operative unit (Tables 1–3).

The surgical patients in category I ($N = 13\,475$) neither had cardiac events in their history nor did the physical examination yield signs indicating cardiac disturbances. Category II ($N = 5464$) comprised all surgical patients who did have cardiac problems in their history. Category III ($N = 10\,523$) comprised the controls of healthy young firemen without any signs of systemic diseases, during their yearly routine fitness check-up required for their profession also during three years (1994–1996).

**Table 1.** Category I: elective non-cardiac surgery without cardiac history ($N = 13\,475$).

| Age range (years) | 21–30 | 31–40 | 41–50 | 51–60 | >60 | Total | Percentage |
|---|---|---|---|---|---|---|---|
| All patients | 867 | 1936 | 2425 | 2841 | 5388 | 13 475 | 100 |
| Previous infarction | 0 | 0 | 1 | 6 | 22 | 29 | 0.21 |
| No sinus | 2 | 2 | 1 | 9 | 294 | 308 | 2.3 |
| >5 PVC/min | 3 | 0 | 6 | 23 | 101 | 133 | 0.9 |
| Left ventricular hypertrophy | 35 | 49 | 46 | 91 | 251 | 472 | 3.5 |
| ST changes | 22 | 52 | 115 | 256 | 1270 | 1715 | 12.7 |
| Bundle branch block | 17 | 28 | 35 | 77 | 496 | 663 | 4.8 |
| WPW syndrome | 3 | 1 | 3 | 4 | 3 | 14 | 0.1 |
| Total | 82 | 132 | 207 | 466 | 2437 | 3334 | 32.0 |
| Percentage | 9.5 | 6.8 | 8.5 | 16.4 | 45.2 | 24.7 | |

**Table 2.** Category II: elective non-cardiac surgery with cardiac history ($N = 5464$).

| Age range (years) | <30 | 31–40 | 41–50 | 51–60 | >60 | Total | Percentage |
|---|---|---|---|---|---|---|---|
| All patients | 93 | 207 | 476 | 947 | 3741 | 5464 | 100 |
| Previous infarction | 0 | 3 | 11 | 38 | 191 | 243 | 4.5 |
| No sinus | 0 | 4 | 9 | 51 | 551 | 613 | 11.2 |
| >5 PVC/min | 0 | 4 | 13 | 9 | 92 | 118 | 2.2 |
| Left ventricular hypertrophy | 1 | 4 | 14 | 47 | 241 | 307 | 5.6 |
| ST changes | 6 | 21 | 79 | 262 | 1690 | 2058 | 37.7 |
| Bundle branch block | 4 | 3 | 7 | 24 | 232 | 270 | 4.9 |
| WPW syndrome | 2 | 2 | 4 | 3 | 5 | 16 | 0.3 |
| Total | 13 | 41 | 137 | 434 | 3002 | 3625 | 79.2 |
| Percentage | 13.9 | 19.8 | 28.8 | 45.8 | 80.2 | 66.3 | |

**Table 3.** Category III: healthy young firemen ($N = 10\,523$).

| Age range (years) | <30 | 31–40 | 41–50 | 51–60 | >60 | Total | Percentage |
|---|---|---|---|---|---|---|---|
| All patients | 3670 | 4131 | 2008 | 667 | 47 | 10 523 | 100 |
| Previous infarction | 0 | 0 | 0 | 1 | 0 | 1 | 0.009 |
| No sinus | 5 | 0 | 0 | 1 | 1 | 7 | 0.06 |
| >5 PVC/min | 14 | 20 | 9 | 6 | 0 | 49 | 0.46 |
| Left ventricular hypertrophy | 27 | 30 | 19 | 7 | 0 | 83 | 0.7 |
| ST changes | 1 | 1 | 3 | 2 | 1 | 8 | 0.076 |
| Bundle branch block | 4 | 12 | 12 | 8 | 0 | 36 | 0.34 |
| WPW syndrome | 7 | 6 | 2 | 0 | 0 | 15 | 0.14 |
| Total | 58 | 69 | 45 | 25 | 2 | 199 | 1.89 |
| Percentage | 1.58 | 1.67 | 2.24 | 3.75 | 4.2 | 1.89 | |

Approximately one-half (48.2%) of the patients scheduled for elective non-cardiac surgery were over 60 years old. The firemen were younger, with only 0.39% of them older than 60 years and 80.3% younger than 40 years.

## INTERPRETATION

Despite no hints of any cardiac events in their history, 32% of our pre-operative patients from category I showed relevant pathological changes in the ECG. The highest percentage of pathological ECG findings was not unexpectedly found in category II of pre-operative patients with known cardiac disturbances (79.2%). Category III, the young healthy firemen, had the lowest rate of pathological findings (1.89%) (Tables 1–3).

The distribution of the subtypes of pathological ECG findings varied among the three categories.

Signs of coronary heart disease with changes of the ST segment were found in 11.2% (category I) and 12.7% (category II) of pre-operative patients, whereas firemen showed ST changes in only 0.076% of all investigations. Signs of previous myocardial infarction were present in 0.21% of category I and in 0.009% of firemen; they were 20 times more frequent, however, in the category with cardiac history (4.5%).

More than five PVC/min, one of the markers used in the cardiac risk index of Goldman et al, were rarely found in category I (0.9%), more frequently in category II (2.2%) and very rarely in category III (0.46%).

A pre-excitation syndrome (WPW or Lown-Ganong-Levine (LGL)) was found rarely and usually in the younger ages in the categories without any known cardiac disturbances and in only 0.3% in the patients with cardiac history.

The fact that the percentage of all relevant pathological ECG findings is increasing with age can be emphasized. Surgical patients over 60 years of age with no cardiac history showed a 45% rate of pre-operative pathological ECG changes and a rate of 80% if previous cardiac events were recorded. There is no discussion about the usefulness of an ECG screening in this age group.

A threshold of age, however, seems to be much more difficult to find. The difference between the age groups (40, 50 or 60 years) of the firemen was small. On the other hand, the surgical patients without any cardiac history and under 40 years of age showed a rate of 7.63% pathological results, equalling 214 patients in 3 years in our data collection. The pathological changes included signs of ventricular hypertrophy as well as bundle branch block or ST changes. Furthermore, it is remarkable that the surgical patients, who apart from their surgical disease felt subjectively healthy, had a higher frequency of relevant pathological ECG than the firemen of the same age. The firemen were a selected group of healthy men with entrance checks and controls. It may seem that the subjective feeling of being 'healthy' is not the same in these two groups.

The most important reason to perform a pre-operative ECG is to rule out a recent myocardial infarction. Kannel and Abbott (1984) reported that 28% of all infarctions were only discovered because of the appearance of ECG changes. This study and others document the clinical importance of pre-operative ECG, which increases with the age of the patient (Medalie and Goldbourt, 1976; Moorman et al, 1985). The presence of a Q wave alone without time-related symptoms of a cardiac event does not represent an alarming sign. However, any Q wave indicates a previous myocardial infarction and serves as a clue to coronary artery disease which is why it must not be underestimated.

Goldman et al (1977) identified two ECG findings that increased the risk of peri-operative cardiac complications. One was a rhythm other than sinus or premature atrial contractions on the last pre-operative ECG, including atrial fibrillation, atrial flutter, junctional rhythm, wandering or electrical pacemaker or atrial tachycardia. Forrest et al (1992) showed an increased peri-operative morbidity and mortality with an higher incidence of atrial fibrillation.

The other important finding was the presence of more than five premature ventricular ectopies per minute (Goldman et al, 1977; Goldman, 1995). Whereas such arrhythmias were documented to be markers of increased peri-operative risk, there is no evidence of a benefit of an anti-arrhythmic therapy. In the diagnosis of arrhythmias auscultation may be helpful, but it is impossible to distinguish between supraventricular or ventricular ectopies or to focus the centre of the pacemaker in eurhythmy (sinus–junctional-wandering pacemaker etc.). Seymour et al (1983) found that left ventricular hypertrophy and ST wave abnormalities were associated with post-operative cardiac complications in elderly women. Von Knorring et al found a correlation between ST abnormalities associated with hypertension as increasing risk factor for post-operative myocardial infarction. Vanik and Davis observed a correlation between the presence of pre-operative and the development of post-operative arrythmias. Bundle branch block, either left or right or bifascicular, has not been identified as an independent risk factor for cardiac complications (Belloci et al, 1980).

Another cardiac disturbance, the WPW syndrome, usually found in younger people, can theoretically cause intraoperative problems (Caramella et al, 1983). Tachycardia is frequent in these individuals; some anti-arrhythmic drugs are contraindicated in the presence of a WPW syndrome. Another reason why it is essential to detect the presence of this so-called pre-excitation syndrome with the help of a pre-operative resting ECG is the fact that most anaesthetic drugs are known to prolong the right artrial refractory period.

However, in all these studies only surgical patients with no or minor cardiac risk who afterwards had surgery were included. Patients for whom surgery was cancelled because of the documented increased cardiac risk were excluded from all peri-operative studies. Therefore the significance of pre-operative ECG changes might have been undervalued by these studies.

In conclusion, the ECG can detect a small group of risk factors that are not always apparent on routine physical examination and history. The control group of healthy firemen with an overall 1.89% incidence of relevant ECG findings showed that ECG screening may be useful even in completely healthy persons of all ages above 20 years. In combination with an exact physical examination and a careful judgement of the findings to prevent hasty decisions due to false-positive results, the resting ECG is a non-invasive, inexpensive and helpful pre-operative test.

## REFERENCES


Belloci F, Santarelli P, Di Gennaro M et al (1980) The risk of cardiac complications in surgical patients with bifascicular block; a clinical and electrophysiologic study in 98 patients. *Chest* **77:** 343–348.

Caramella JP, Malbenzin S, Couderc E et al (1983) Anaesthesia in patient with the ventricular pre-excitation syndrome. *Canadian Anaesthesiology Society Journal* **30:** 185–190.

Eagle KE, Brundage BH, Chaitman BR et al (1996) Guidelines for perioperative cardiovascular evaluation for non-cardiac surgery. *Journal of the American College of Cardiology* **7(4):** 910–948.

Elston RA & Taylor DJ (1984) The preoperative ECG. *Lancet* **1:** 349.

Forrest JB, Rehder K, Cahalan M & Goldsmith CH (1992) Multicenter study of general anesthesia. *Anesthesiology* **76:** 3–15.

*Goldberger AL & O'Kinsky M (1986) Utility of the routine electrocardiogram before surgery and on general hospital admission. *Annals of Internal Medicine* **105:** 552–557.

*Goldman L (1995) Cardiac risk in noncardiac surgery: an update. *Anaesthesia and Analgesia* **80:** 810–820.

*Goldman L, Caldera DL, Nussbaum SR et al (1977) Multifactorial index of cardiac risk in noncardiac surgical procedures. *New England Journal of Medicine* **297:** 845–850.

Kannel WB & Abbott RD (1984) Incidence and prognosis of unrecognized myocardial infarction: an update of the Framingham study. *New England Journal of Medicine* **311:** 1144–1147.

Von Knorring J (1981) Postoperative myocardial infarction: a prospective study in a risk group of surgical patients. *Surgery* **90:** 55–60.

List WF (1984) Die präoperative Anästhesieambulanz. In *Klinische Anästhesie Current Reviews*, vol. 2. Graz: Akademische Druck- und Verlagsgesellschaft.

Medalie JH & Goldbourt U (1976) Unrecognized myocardial infarction. Five year incidence, mortality and risk factors. *Annals of Internal Medicine* **84:** 526–531.

Moorman JR, Hlatky MA, Eddy DM & Wagner GS (1985) The yield of the admission electrocardiogram: a study in a general medical service. *Annals of Internal Medicine* **103:** 590–595.

*Prause G (1994) The preoperative outpatient clinic in Graz: the first 15 years. *Anaesthesist* **43:** 223–228.

Prause G, Gombotz H, Rehak P & List WF (1990) The preoperative clinic—a probable use for a personal computer. *Anaesthesist* **39:** 186–190.

Roizen MF (1986) Routine preoperative evaluation. In Miller RD (ed.) *Anesthesia*, pp 225–253. New York: Churchill Livingstone.

Seymour DG, Pringle R & MacLennan WJ (1983) The role of the routine preoperative electrocardiogram in the elderly patient. *Age and Ageing* **12:** 97–104.

Vanik PE & Davis HS (1986) Cardiac arrhythmias during halothane anesthesia. *Anaesth Analg* **47:** 229–307.

# 3

# Pre-operative screening for elective surgery

WOLFGANG F. DICK FRCA

Director
*International Trauma Anaesthesia Critical Care Society*

Vice-chairman
*European Resuscitation Council*

Hon. Secretary
*World Association of Disaster and Emergency Medicine*

President
*German Association of Critical Care Medicine (DIVI)*

Chairman, Department of Anaesthesiology
*Klinik für Anästhesiologie, Klinikum der Universität Mainz, Langenbeckstr. 1, 55131 Mainz, Germany*

The primary goal of pre-operative evaluation is to assess adequately the patient's pre-operative condition and to diagnose and possibly to treat disturbances and diseases which may be of relevance to the course of anaesthesia, surgery and the post-operative period. A pertinent medical history and a physical examination by an experienced anaesthetist are compulsory. A minimal set of tests should be carried out in all patients. The results obtained from these tests were very abnormal in a variety of studies; the information was not always apparent from the history and the examination although it was of relevance to anaesthesia and the post-operative period. Further laboratory tests such as haematocrit and blood glucose and potassium ($K^+$) concentrations should only be ordered if indicated on the basis of the history and the examination. This small set of tests seems to be justified for the following reasons:

- to identify unexpected risk factors not apparent from the history and the examination;
- to avoid additional costs resulting from deferring a case due to incomplete tests;
- to avoid medicolegal consequences of a possibly incomplete pre-operative evaluation;
- to protect patients from unnecessary invasive investigations.

**Key words:** pre-operative evaluation; medical history; physical examination; complications; X-ray; electrocardiogram; laboratory tests.

The primary goal of pre-operative evaluation is to assess adequately the patient's pre-operative condition and to diagnose and possibly to treat disturbances and diseases which may be of relevance to the course of anaesthesia, surgery and the post-operative period (Dick et al, 1978; Osswald et al, 1985; Duncan and Cohen, 1987; Goldman, 1987; Turnbull and Buck, 1987; Roizen, 1988; Feddersen, 1990; Perez et al, 1995). In


ISBN 0-7020-2536-4
0950-3501/98/030349 + 23 $12.00/00

recent years, intensive efforts have been made to identify risk factors which might contribute to unexpected morbidity or mortality during and after the course of anaesthesia. Now that our goal of minimizing morbidity and mortality has almost been achieved, some critical voices are heard (Hubbel et al, 1985; Roizen, 1988; Fischer, 1990; Gold et al, 1992; Archer et al, 1993; Mantha et al, 1994; Lee et al, 1997; Vogt and Henson, 1997) claiming that we might be doing too much to protect our patients from harm resulting from the interference between pre-existing diseases and medication on the one hand and anaesthesia, including the post-operative course, on the other. The cost–benefit ratio may be imbalanced and patients might even be harmed if subjected to non-indicated invasive procedures. In order to separate the wheat from the chaff, and to come to evidence-based recommendations, we need to answer a number of specific questions.

1. Should the minimal requirements for pre-operative evaluation merely consist of the medical history and the physical examination?
2. What does an anaesthesia-related medical history comprise?
3. What does an anaesthesia-related physical examination include?
4. What is the percentage of unknown disturbances and diseases which cannot be identified on the basis of the medical history and a thorough physical examination alone (without using laboratory tests, electrocardiogram (ECG), X-ray etc.)?
5. What do abnormal results imply?
6. Should abnormal results always be rechecked before any conclusions are drawn, considering that many of these results are abnormal in the first instance and tend to return to normal levels later?
7. When are abnormal results of ECG, X-ray or laboratory parameters relevant to anaesthesia? Are they related to intra- or post-operative complications?
8. Are we likely to harm our patients by performing too many pre-operative investigations and by drawing doubtful therapeutic conclusions on the basis of abnormal results?
9. What is the ratio of the per diem cost of deferring a case to that of a routine pre-operative programme?

## THE PRIMARY GOAL OF PRE-OPERATIVE EVALUATION

The primary goal of pre-operative evaluation is to assess adequately the patient's pre-operative condition and to diagnose and possibly to treat disturbances and diseases which may be of relevance to anaesthesia, surgery and the post-operative course. The primary outcome parameters are morbidity, the rate and type of complications, the length of intensive care unit (ICU) and hospital stay, unexpected admission to the ICU, and mortality. Pre-operative test results may be correlated with these parameters.

Most studies agree that there are two types of neither invasive nor expensive evaluations which should be routinely performed in every patient pre-operatively:

1. a pertinent medical history and
2. a physical examination.

## Medical history

As anaesthesia affects almost all organ functions, an anaesthesia-related medical history should concentrate on the following organ systems: central nervous (stroke, tumour etc.), respiratory (asthma, chronic obstructive pulmonary disease (COPD) etc.), cardiovascular (myocardial infarction, hypertension, dysrhythmias etc.) and metabolic organ (diabetes, malignancy etc.) systems; 'Most valuable information about ischaemic heart disease can be derived from a meticulous patient history including details of other risk factors such as organ dysfunctions and metabolic disorders and of their medical treatment. Anything suspicious in this should lead to a careful and more detailed diagnosis in order to quantify the degree of the respective disease.' (Feddersen, 1990).

The medical history should include questions on liver and renal problems, bleeding disorders, present complaints such as backache, current and previous medication, anaphylactic events, transfusions, previous anaesthetic exposures and surgical interventions, smoking habits etc. However, only those factors of a medical history can be considered for anaesthesia which are reported by the patient or are asked for by the anaesthesiologist (Figure 1).

This is absolutely crucial in patients (generally older ones) who claim never to have undergone treatment in the relevant hospital, thus precluding a search for previous records. Furthermore, medicolegal aspects may come into play here; in some countries jurisdiction requires that the responsible physician must check whether a patient has previously been admitted to a hospital, be it as an out-patient or in-patient and regardless of whether the patient denies ever having undergone treatment there. This procedure may be further complicated by the fact that even university hospital computer systems may not be sufficiently advanced to provide this information at night-time or on holidays.

A pertinent medical history should include questions on complaints, central nervous system disorders, respiratory disorders, cardiovascular diseases, metabolic disorders, liver–renal diseases, medication, anaphylactic reactions, bleeding–coagulation abnormalities, previous transfusions, previous anaesthetics, smoking habits, etc.

## The physical examination

A physical examination must be anaesthesia related and should include

- a talk with the patient to check the mental status,
- an inspection of the head and neck,
- an inspection of the oral and nasal cavity for possible airway problems,
- an inspection of the sites for venous and arterial accesses,
- determination of the status of the vertebral column, particularly if a spinal or epidural anaesthesia (EDA) is planned,
- auscultation and percussion of heart and lungs,
- blood pressure checks (possibly on both arms),

**englisch** A13

Department of Anaesthesiology

# Patient Information and Medical History Form for Adults

**Aufklärungs- und Anamnesebogen für Erwachsene**

Address of Patient
Patientenadresse

## Please read this soon and answer the questions

**Hold yourself ready for a conversation with the anaesthetist one day before the operation!**

## To the patient:

Painful examinations and treatments are performed regularly under anaesthesia (loss of pain sensation).

The anaesthetist has the responsibility of deterring pain and maintaining the vital functions (particularly respiration and circulation) during the surgical operation. His cooperation with the physician performing the operation serves to ensure patient safety.

Various procedures are used in anaesthetizing the patient:

## General Anaesthesia

involves a loss of consciousness and sensation to pain in the entire body. At the beginning of the anaesthesia, the patient falls into a quiet, sleep-like state which is maintained to the very end.

Following an injection (pre-medication), the anaesthesia is generally induced by injecting an anaesthetic agent adequate for short operations (intravenous short-acting anaesthetics). For operations of longer duration, the injection is repeated (intravenous anaesthesia) or the anaesthesia is prolonged by using a gaseous agent inhaled over a mask or an endotracheal tube.

In anaesthetic procedures using a mask, the patient receives oxygen and anaesthetics through a mask that covers his mouth and nose.

In anaesthetic procedures using intubation the patient receives oxygen and anaesthetics through a tube inserted into the trachea (wind pipe) after he has fallen asleep. Use of the endotracheal tube permits a high degree of safety in breathing and protects the lungs from the consequences of vomiting. By the addition of muscle relaxants, the surgical conditions can be improved and the amount of anaesthetics reduced.

## Local Anaesthesia

entails a loss of sensation to pain in certain regions of the body **(regional or conduction anaesthesia)** or in the immediate area of the operation (local anaesthesia).

**Brachial-plexus anaesthesia,** for example, causes a loss of the pain sensation in one arm only. **Spinal and peridural/epidural anaesthesia** prevents perception of stimuli in certain regions by blocking the pain nerves leading to the spinal cord. At a certain point of the spinal column, the anaesthetic is injected into the area around the pain nerves. The puncture is painless because the puncture area is numbed beforehand.

## Selection of the anaesthetic procedure

Every type of anaesthesia has its advantages and disadvantages. We recommend the procedure which is

Von der Allgemeinen Deutschen Patienten-Organisation (A. D. P. O.) überprüft und empfohlen.

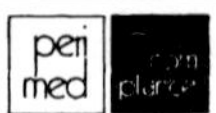



**Figure 1 (see pages 344–347).** Example of a patient information and medical history form. Reproduced with permission from Perimed-Compliance, Erlangen, Germany.

most suited for the operation planned and involves the least discomfort.

## No surgery is without risk

Severe accidents associated with anaesthesia, such as cardiac arrest, are very rare, even for patients in poor general condition.

Modern **General Anaesthesia**, with its exact dosage, the combination of various anaesthetic agents, and the use of respirators makes it possible to keep the respiration, the circulation and other vital bodily functions under control. In order to prevent complications, these functions are monitored during the entire anaesthesia. In cooperation with the performing surgeon, the position on the operating table is constantly supervised in order to avoid injuries to nerves (dysaesthesia, paralysis) that could result from pressure or strain.

**Local Anaesthesia** places little strain on the organism. Contrary to the apprehensions of many patients, injuries to nerves are extremely rare, even in spinal and peridural/epidural anaesthesia.

## Please follow these instructions

in order to avoid aspiration accidents (inhalation of vomit).

Do not eat or drink anything 6–8 hours prior to the operation and do not smoke during these 6 hours.

Take out removable parts of teeth (artificial teeth, dentures) and contact lenses. Remove all make-up, nail polish, earrings, rings, necklaces, wigs and toupees before the operation.

## Please inform us

As with any surgery, the strains of anaesthesia and its hazards are contingent on the circumstances of the individual case. Of particular importance are the type and severity of the disorder and any previous illnesses or accompanying diseases, general condition of health, and daily habits.

The following questions are designed to cover all possible risks and thereby assure the greatest possible safety. The reason for the large number of questions is that we want to avoid even rare and relatively insignificant risks (eg. injuries to teeth during intubation, irritation to veins, voice box injuries, nausea, and vomiting).

In the column "Other", please give any information you consider important.

If you need assistance in answering these questions, please ask your nurse or anaesthetist.

## Medical History Record

Fragen zur Anamnese

Age:__________ height:______ centimeters
Alter: Jahre Größe cm

Weight:______________ kilograms
Gewicht: kg

**no = nein/yes = ja**

1. What is your profession?
1. Welchen Beruf üben Sie aus?

______________________________

2. Have you been in a physician's care lately? ☐ no yes ☐
For which disease(s):
2. Befanden Sie sich in letzter Zeit in ärztlicher Behandlung? Wegen welcher Erkrankungen:

______________________________

______________________________

3. Are you pregnant? ☐ no yes ☐
3. Besteht eine Schwangerschaft?

4. Were you taking medication before being sent to the hospital? ☐ no yes ☐
Which medication? Also list pain-killers, sleeping-tablets, sedatives, laxatives, contraceptives (birth control pills)
4. Nehmen Sie zur Zeit Medikamente ein? Welche? Geben Sie auch Schmerz-, Schlaf-, Beruhigungs-, Abführmittel, Ovulationshemmer („Antibabypille") an.

______________________________

______________________________

5. Any previous operations (eg. gall-bladder operation 1974, inguinal hernia operation 1978)
5. Frühere Operationen (z. B. „Galle 1974", „Leistenbruch 1978")

a) ______________________ year ________
b) ______________________ year ________
c) ______________________ year ________
d) ______________________ year ________
a)–d) im Jahre

Was there anything unusual in the anaesthesia? ☐ no yes ☐
What?
Ergaben sich bei der Anästhesie Besonderheiten? Welche?

______________________________

Have any blood relatives had complications from anaesthetization? ☐ no yes ☐
Kam es bei Blutsverwandten zu Zwischenfällen im Zusammenhang mit einer Anästhesie?

6. Did you ever had any blood transfusion? ☐ no yes ☐
Did complications result from that transfusion? ☐ no yes ☐
6. Haben Sie schon einmal eine Bluttransfusion bekommen? Ergaben sich dabei Komplikationen?

**Are you aware of now having or having had any of the following diseases?**
**Ist Ihnen bekannt, ob Sie an einer der folgenden Krankheiten leiden oder litten?**

7. Muscular disease or muscular weakness? ☐ no yes ☐
7. Muskelerkrankungen und Muskelschwäche?

**no = nein/yes = ja**

Having now or having had any of your blood relatives such disease? ☐ no yes ☐

Gab oder gibt es eine solche Erkrankung bei Ihren Blutsverwandten?

8. Heart disease, eg. heart attack (myocardial infarction), angina pectoris, organic disease of the heart (cardiac defect), difficulties in breathing when climbing stairs, myocarditis (inflammation of the cardiac muscle), cardiac arrhythmias? ☐ no yes ☐

8. Herzerkrankungen (z. B. Herzinfarkt, Angina pectoris, Herzfehler, Atemnot beim Treppensteigen, Herzmuskelentzündung, Herzrhythmusstörungen)?

9. Circulatory or vascular diseases (eg. circulation disturbances, varicose veins, thrombosis, high blood pressure, low blood pressure)? ☐ no yes ☐

9. Kreislauf- und Gefäßerkrankungen (z. B. Durchblutungsstörungen, Krampfadern, Thrombose, zu hoher oder zu niedriger Blutdruck)?

10. Lung or respiratory tract diseases (eg. tuberculosis, pulmonary emphysema, pneumoconiosis, pneumonia, asthma, chronic bronchitis)? ☐ no yes ☐

10. Lungen- und Atemwegserkrankungen (z. B. Tuberkulose, Staublunge, Lungenentzündung, Lungenblähung, Asthma, chronische Bronchitis)?

11. Diseases of the liver (eg. jaundice, hepatic induration)? ☐ no yes ☐

11. Lebererkrankungen (z. B. Gelbsucht, Leberverhärtung)?

12. Kidney disease (eg. inflammation of kidney (nephritis), kidney stones)? ☐ no yes ☐

12. Nierenerkrankungen (z. B. Nierenentzündung, Nierensteine)?

13. Metabolic disorders such as diabetes, fructose intolerance (intolerance of fruit)? ☐ no yes ☐

13. Stoffwechselerkrankungen, z. B. Zuckerkrankheit, Fruchtzuckerunverträglichkeit (Unverträglichkeit von Obst)?

14. Diseases of the thyroid gland (eg. goitre)? ☐ no yes ☐

14. Schilddrüsenerkrankungen (z. B. Kropf)?

15. Eye diseases (eg. glaucoma)? ☐ no yes ☐

15. Augenerkrankungen (z. B. grüner Star)?

16. Nervous disorders (eg. epilepsy, paralysis)? ☐ no yes ☐

16. Nervenleiden (z. B. Krampfleiden, Lähmungen)?

17. Have you received medical treatment for any psychiatric disorders (eg. depressions)? ☐ no yes ☐

17. Gemütsleiden (z. B. Depressionen)?

18. Diseases of the skeletal system (eg. injuries of the spinal column, diseases of the joints)? ☐ no yes ☐

18. Erkrankungen des Skelettsystems (z. B. Wirbelsäulenschäden, Gelenkserkrankungen)?

19. Blood diseases or coagulation disorders (eg. hemorrhagic tendencies, nose bleeds)? ☐ no yes ☐

19. Bluterkrankungen oder Blutgerinnungsstörungen (z. B. Neigung zu Blutergüssen, Nasenbluten)?

20. Allergies (eg. hay fever, hypersensitivity to certain foods, medications, or adhesive tapes)? ☐ no yes ☐
Which?

**no = nein/yes = ja**

20. Allergien (z. B. Heuschnupfen, Überempfindlichkeit gegen Nahrungsmittel, Medikamente, Pflaster)? Welche?

________________________________

21. Do you suffer from any disease which is not listed? ☐ no yes ☐
Which?

21. Leiden Sie an einer anderen, nicht aufgeführten Erkrankung? Welche?

________________________________

22. Do you wear dentures (crown teeth, jacket crowns, dental bridges, removable dentures)? ☐ no yes ☐

22. Tragen Sie Zahnersatz (Stiftzähne, Jacketkronen, Zahnbrücken, herausnehmbare Prothesen)?

Do you have any loose teeth? ☐ no yes ☐

Haben Sie lockere Zähne?

________________________________

Dental status (has to be filled in by the physician):

| 4 | 3 | 2 | 1 | 1 | 2 | 3 | 4 |
|---|---|---|---|---|---|---|---|
| 4 | 3 | 2 | 1 | 1 | 2 | 3 | 4 |

× = missing tooth s = teeth cleaned up
O = loose tooth ns = teeth not cleaned up
– = denture

Zahnstatus (wird vom Arzt ausgefüllt)
× = fehlender Zahn, s = saniertes Gebiß
O = lockerer Zahn, ns = nicht saniertes Gebiß
– = Prothese

Habits:

Lebensgewohnheiten:

23. Do you smoke regularly? ☐ no yes ☐

23. Rauchen Sie regelmäßig?

24. Do you drink alcohol on a regular basis? ☐ no yes ☐

24. Trinken Sie regelmäßig Alkohol?

25. Are you used to a special medication? ☐ no yes ☐

25. Sind Sie an bestimmte Medikamente gewöhnt?

26. Do you wear a hearing aid? ☐ no yes ☐

26. Tragen Sie ein Hörgerät?

Other (eg. accidents, preexisting disorders not indicated in this form, special professional conditions):

Sonstige Besonderheiten: (z. B. Unfälle, nicht aufgeführte Vorerkrankungen, besondere berufliche Verhältnisse):

________________________________

## Please ask

the physician about anything having to do with anaesthesia that might be of interest to you. At your request, he will give you all informations concerning any rare and very exceptional risks.

Measures to prepare for surgery, such during surgery (e.g. artificial lowering of blood pressure, infusions, blood transfusions, central vein catheters) and after it (e.g. in the intensive care ward) are not totally free of risks either. Thus a blood transfusion might cause an infection with the hepatitis virus and very rarely with HIV (AIDS). An autotransfusion avoids such risks, it is not always possible, though.

## Affirmation of consent

Einwilligungserklärung

Mr./Mrs.______________________discussed with me today the anaesthetic procedure planned, based on the results of the preliminary examinations and on my answers to the above questions. I understood the explanations and was able to ask any questions which were of interest to me, especially about the procedure, its advantages and disadvantages, special risks involved and possible secondary operations and complementary treatment (eg. artificially lowering the blood pressure, infusions, blood transfusions, central vein catheter, anaesthetic post-operative treatment).

Herr/Frau __________ hat mit mir heute anhand der Ergebnisse der Voruntersuchungen und meiner Antworten zu den vorstehenden Fragen ein Aufklärungsgespräch über das bei mir vorgesehene Anästhesieverfahren geführt. Ich habe die Aufklärung verstanden und konnte alle mich interessierenden Fragen stellen, insbesondere nach der Art des Verfahrens, seinen Vor- und Nachteilen, nach etwaigen Nebeneingriffen und ergänzenden Behandlungsmaßnahmen (z. B. künstliche Blutdrucksenkung, Infusionen, Bluttransfusionen, zentraler Venenkatheter, anästhesiologische Nachbehandlung) sowie nach den damit verbundenen speziellen Risiken.

I have no further questions ☐ **or**
Ich habe keine weiteren Fragen. Oder

Please indicate the questions or cross out these line

Bitte die Fragen bezeichnen oder diese Zeile durchstreichen

I have the following questions:
Ich habe folgende weitere Fragen:

______________________________

______________________________

Physician's comments about patient consultation

(e.g. choice of anaesthesia procedure, factors increasing the risk, probability of blood transfusion becoming necessary, donation of patient's own blood)

Ärztlicher Vermerk zum Aufklärungsgespräch (z. B. Wahl des Betäubungsverfahrens, risikoerhöhende Umstände, Wahrscheinlichkeit einer Bluttransfusion, Eigenblutspende)

______________________________

______________________________

I give my consent to the intended operation/examination
Ich willige ein, daß die geplante Operation/Untersuchung:

Please give detailed description of intended operation:

______________________________

under anaesthesia ☐ under regional anaesthesia ☐
in Narkose in Regionalanästhesie ausgeführt wird.

I also consent to the preparatory and accompanying anaesthetic treatment, including the additional secondary operations. I agree to any medically indicated changes and prolongations of anaesthesia and to any blood transfusion that might become necessary.

Possible restrictions of consent (eg. for certain anaesthesia procedures or secondary operations)

Ich willige weiter in die vorbereitende und begleitende anästhesiologische Behandlung einschließlich der dazu erforderlichen Nebeneingriffe ein. Mit medizinisch angezeigten Änderungen und Erweiterungen der Anästhesie sowie einer evtl. erforderlichen Bluttransfusion bin ich einverstanden. Vermerk über etwaige Beschränkungen der Einwilligung (z. B. hinsichtlich bestimmter Anästhesieverfahren oder von Nebeneingriffen)

______________________________

______________________________

______________________________

Date______________
Datum:

signature of physician
Unterschrift des Arztes

signature of patient or guardian
Unterschrift des Patienten bzw. des Sorgeberechtigten

---

## Instructions for ambulatory operations:

Hinweise für ambulante Eingriffe:

In your own interest please inform the physician if you have had anything to eat or drink 6 hours before the operation.
Remember that you will not be able to operate any vehicle immediately after the anaesthesia. Have your relatives or a taxi pick you up and drive you home after you have been released from the physician's care. Due to secondary effects of the anaestesia, you may not drive, work at machines and not drink alcohol during the following 24 hours.

Date:______________
Datum:

I confirm that I have been made aware of these instructions:

patient's signature
Unterschrift des Patienten

- palpation of the liver,
- check for possible pretibial or other oedema and
- investigation of motility and flexibility of extremities to exclude the possibility of anaesthesia-related post-operative nerve palsies.

## DATA FROM STUDIES CARRIED OUT BY OUR OWN GROUP

- What is the benefit of an anaesthesia-related medical history and physical examination alone if no ECGs, X-rays or laboratory parameters are obtained?
- How many undetected disturbances and diseases may be overlooked and how many may cause complications during and after anaesthesia, if a full set of technical and laboratory investigations is not carried out routinely in any patient undergoing diagnostic and/or therapeutic interventions in general and/or regional anaesthesia?

Any patient with a carefully determined anaesthesia-related medical history and physical status will benefit if X-rays and repeated blood withdrawals are avoided. Roizen (1994) found that a chest X-ray was ordered without indication in almost 64% of 606 patients; in three of these patients, who showed some radiographic pathology, invasive investigations were carried out without any abnormal results. A high percentage of chest X-rays ordered by an anaesthesiologist were never looked at. The German Supreme Court (Kellerer, 1991) recently took a decision which clearly stated that a physician who orders or performs X-rays which are not strictly indicated and balanced against their need can be sued for malpractice.

In order to answer the question of how many unknown and relevant disorders and diseases might be overlooked if only a medical history is obtained and a physical examination is performed, the results of two of our own studies and those obtained by several other investigators will be examined. The design of the studies required that only the medical history was taken and a physical examination was carried out. However, without the knowledge of the responsible anaesthesiologist the results were controlled by routine checks of chest X-rays, ECGs and laboratory tests and subsequently related to outcome in terms of complications or possible mortality.

### How many patients had abnormal test results despite an unremarkable medical history?

One hundred and six out of 379 patients included in a prospective study (Christian et al, 1988) had an unremarkable medical history; 14% of patients, however, showed abnormal ECGs, 22.6% abnormal chest X-rays and 17.9% abnormal laboratory tests; 8.5% or 3.8% of tests, respectively, were of relevance to anaesthesia, while only 2% of the abnormal ECG results could be related to peri-operative complications (Table 1). Thus, a variety of unexpected results would have been missed if only the medical history had been taken.

**Table 1.** Incidence of abnormal test results in patients with non-contributory medical history.

| Test type | Abnormal (%) | Relevant to anaesthesia (%) | Related to complications (%) |
|---|---|---|---|
| ECG | 14.1 | 8.5 | 1.9 |
| X-ray | 22.6 | 3.8 | 0.0 |
| Laboratory tests | 17.9 | 0.0 | 0.0 |

## How many patients had normal results based on the physical examination but showed abnormal test results?

The results of a meticulous physical examination were normal in 154 of 379 patients. Approximately 17% of patients had abnormal ECGs, 28% had abnormal chest X-rays and 19% abnormal laboratory tests. However, only 9% of the abnormal ECGs and 2% of the X-rays were of relevance to anaesthesia and only 2% of the abnormal ECGs could be related to peri-operative complications (Table 2).

**Table 2.** Incidence of abnormal test results in patients with normal physical examination.

| Test type | Abnormal (%) | Relevant to anaesthesia (%) | Related to complications (%) |
|---|---|---|---|
| ECG | 16.8 | 9.1 | 1.9 |
| Chest X-ray | 27.9 | 1.9 | 0.0 |
| Laboratory tests | 18.8 | 0.0 | 0.0 |

## Abnormal test results in patients with normal medical history and physical examination

Although the medical history and physical examination were both normal in 106 of the 379 study patients, 14% of abnormal ECGs, 22.6% of abnormal chest X-rays and 18% of abnormal laboratory tests would have been missed. Nevertheless, only 8.5% of abnormal ECGs and 3.8% of abnormal chest X-rays were of relevance to anaesthesia and only 2% of the abnormal ECGs could be related to complications (Table 3).

Surprisingly, independently of whether the measures were essential or not, the responsible anaesthetist ordered far more additional investigations than required on the basis of the results of the medical history and his or her examination. Although only 273 patients showed some pathology in the medical history and physical examination, additional laboratory tests were

**Table 3.** Incidence of abnormal test results in patients with normal medical history and physical examination.

| Test type | Abnormal (%) | Relevant to anaesthesia (%) | Related to complications (%) |
|---|---|---|---|
| ECG | 14.1 | 8.5 | 1.9 |
| Chest X-ray | 22.6 | 3.8 | 0.0 |
| Laboratory tests | 17.9 | 0.0 | 0.0 |

ordered in 100% of the cases, ECGs in 93% and chest X-rays in 78% (Table 4).

What might have been the reasons for these prima facie unjustified tests? From the premise that it is in the interest of a given patient not to be put at risk, for example as a result of intra- and peri-operative complications, only those tests would have been justified which were shown to be of potential relevance to anaesthesia and could be related to complications.

**Table 4.** Requested tests by the responsible anaesthetist (rarely) based on medical history and physical examination.

| Medical history or physical examination remarkable | Test type | Requested (%) | Abnormal (%) |
|---|---|---|---|
| 72% | ECG | 93 | 42 |
| | X-ray | 76 | 57 |
| | Laboratory | 100 | 31 |
| | Pulmonary function test | 4 | 53 |
| | Consultation | 23 | 58 |
| | Other | 2 | 62 |

In summary, if merely the results of the medical history and the physical examination carried out by an experienced anaesthesiologist had been considered, the following would have been missed:

- 8.5% of abnormal ECGs of relevance to anaesthesia and associated with complications and
- no abnormal X-rays or laboratory tests with relevance to anaesthesia and associated with complications.

Thus, the majority of the ECGs and all X-rays and laboratory tests which were ordered in patients with an unremarkable medical history and normal physical examination were unjustified.

## Considerations in elderly patients

It is known that the number of abnormal results for both history and physical examination increase with age (Table 5). Additional investigations reflected the results of a contributory medical history and an abnormal result from physical examination (Table 6).

**Table 5.** Incidence of abnormal results on physical examination related to the incidence of pre-existing diseases and medication detected by the medical history.

| | Medical history | | |
|---|---|---|---|
| Age (years) | Pre-existing disease (%) | Pre-existing medication (%) | Abnormal physical examination (%) |
| ≤29 | 34 | 27 | 10 |
| 30–39 | 38 | 31 | 26 |
| 40–49 | 60 | 39 | 47 |
| 50–59 | 79 | 64 | 66 |
| 60–69 | 93 | 77 | 82 |
| ≥70 | 97 | 88 | 87 |

**Table 6.** Incidence of abnormal test results in relation to the incidence of pre-existing diseases.

| Age (years) | Pre-existing disease (%) | Abnormal ECG (%) | Abnormal X-ray (%) | Abnormal laboratory tests (%) |
|---|---|---|---|---|
| ≤29 | 34 | 5 | – | 5 |
| 30–39 | 38 | 2.5 | 2.5 | 14 |
| 40–49 | 60 | 10 | 6 | 25 |
| 50–59 | 79 | 16 | 10 | 37 |
| 60–69 | 93 | 34 | 15 | 42 |
| ≥70 | 97 | 41 | 26 | 46 |

It is, however, surprising to note that, despite the presence of pre-existing diseases, these diseases were expressed in only 30–40% of the younger age groups by abnormal ECGs and X-rays in 2.5–5% of patients. In contrast to patients whose medical history and physical examination were without pathological findings, there was a significant intra- and post-operative complication rate in patients with a pathological medical history and physical examination. Complications occurred in roughly 30–50% of the patients with pathological ECG, X-ray or laboratory test findings and almost all intraoperative complications were of relevance to anaesthesia; of the post-operative complications only 30% were important for patient recovery. The latter were associated with age, pre-existing diseases and medication as well as with abnormal results of the physical examination (Tables 7 and 8).

In 10 out of 35 patients with intraoperative haemodynamic complications abnormal results were observed on the pre-operative ECG (four cases) and the chest X-ray (one case); complications were suspected on the basis of the medical history and/or physical examination in five cases (Table 9).

**Table 7.** Incidence of intra- and post-operative complications related to the frequency of pre-existing diseases.

| Age (years) | Pre-existing disease (%) | Complications (%) | |
|---|---|---|---|
| | | Intraoperative | Post-operative |
| ≤29 | 34 | 7.0 | 2.5 |
| 30–39 | 38 | 7.0 | 2.5 |
| 40–49 | 60 | 14.0 | 5.5 |
| 50–59 | 79 | 18.5 | 10.0 |
| 60–69 | 93 | 24.0 | 12.0 |
| ≥70 | 97 | 23.0 | 14.5 |

**Table 8.** Incidence of complications in relation to pre-existing diseases and abnormal test results.

| | Rate | Intraoperative $N=65$ (17%) | Post-operative $N=33$ (8.7%) |
|---|---|---|---|
| Pre-existing diseases (none) | 72 | 19 (11) | 10 (5) |
| Abnormal physical examination (normal) | 59 | 20 (13) | 12 (4) |
| Abnormal ECG (normal) | 41 | 17 (17) | 12 (6) |
| Abnormal X-ray (normal) | 49 | 19 (17) | 10 (8) |
| Abnormal laboratory tests (normal) | 31 | 18 (16) | 13 (7) |

**Table 9.** Peri-operative complications ($N = 48$) related to pre-operative evaluation.

| | | | |
|---|---|---|---|
| Intraoperative | Haemodynamic | $N = 35$ | 29% |
| Post-operative | Cardiorespiratory | $N = 13$ | 69% |

In the 13 patients with post-operative cardiorespiratory events the pre-operative ECG (two cases) and X-ray (two cases) were abnormal, while the history and examination showed cardiorespiratory abnormalities in another five patients.

## DATA OBTAINED BY OTHER STUDIES

When comparing our results in a selected group of patients (who were, however, representative for the patient population admitted to our hospital to undergo surgery) with results reported by other authors and those obtained by a retrospective study in 2500 patients performed by our group some years ago (Altemeyer et al, 1984), it becomes apparent that the number of abnormal test results in patients with a normal history and physical examination is significantly higher in the prospective studies than in the retrospective ones.

### Electrocardiograms

On the basis of calculations made by Diamond and Forrester (1979) regarding the need for a pre-operative ECG, Paraskos (1992) arrived at interesting values for the likelihood of the development of coronary artery disease (CAD) with or without ‘non-anginal’ chest pain (Table 10). Kilian et al (1987), List et al (1985), and Mehrkens et al (1987) reported unsuspected ECG results in 2.1% or 4.1% of patients (compared with 14.1% in our prospective study).

It is, however, important to note that only abnormal test results likely to be missed exerted an influence on peri-operative complications. In a retrospective investigation Gold et al (1992) described the routine performance of an ECG as possibly useful in six out of 751 patients. On the basis of the results obtained by this study Gold et al question the usefulness of the routine performance of pre-operative ECG (Table 11). This hypothesis has been confirmed by findings reported by Hyman (1990) and Feddersen (1990). In a multicentre study Perez et al (1995) observed 5.6% unexpected

**Table 10.** Likelihood of coronary artery disease in relation to age (Diamond and Forrester, 1979; Paraskos, 1992).

| | Likelihood (%) | |
|---|---|---|
| Age (years) | Male | Female |
| 40–49 | 5.5 | 1 |
| 50–59 | 9.7 | 5.5 |

**Table 11.** Incidence of abnormal electrocardiograms in relation to relevance and complications.

| | Abnormal (%) | Relevant to anaesthesia (%) | Relevant to complications (%) |
|---|---|---|---|
| Gold et al (1992) | 37–62 | 11.6 | 1.6 |
| Christian et al (1990) | 14 | 8.5 | 1.9 |
| Johnson et al (1988) | 44 | | |
| Vogt and Henson (1997) | | 80 | |
| Perez et al (1995) | 5.6 | 0.46 | |
| McKee and Scott (1987) | 30 | 2 | 23 |

abnormal ECGs, although anaesthetic management had to be changed in only 0.46% of patients. When a small number of the tests showing abnormal results were repeated, one out of five controversial findings was shown to be normal. Callaghan et al (1995) observed five abnormal ECGs in patients older than 50 years with no known risk factors while even higher incidence rates were reported by other investigators. The fact that some studies greatly underestimate the importance of abnormal findings is emphasized by a comparison of the results obtained by our retrospective and prospective studies which also show a higher incidence of abnormal findings in the prospective than in the retrospective investigation. The available data lead to the conclusion that retrospective data underestimate the incidence of abnormal tests. It is, however, open to question (Table 12) whether the retrospective data imply the presence of a greater number of risk factors than prospective data.

**Table 12.** Pre-operative evaluation: abnormal history and examination (Christian et al, 1988).

| | Prospective (%) | Retrospective (%) |
|---|---|---|
| Overall abnormal | 59 | 44 |
| ECG | 56 | 15 |
| X-ray | 65 | 6.5 |
| Laboratory tests | 41 | 10 |

## Chest X-rays

Similar age-independent results were reported for chest X-rays (Table 13). Perez et al (1995) described 22.5% abnormal chest X-rays, 8.6% of which were unexpected (almost identical to our results), although only 0.56% led to changes in the management of the case. In a prospective study in 517 patients Hartung (1990) found that some patients with a normal history and physical examination had an abnormal chest X-ray. Similar findings were reported by other authors (Petterson and Janover, 1977; Haubek and Gold, 1978; Seymour et al, 1982; Törnebrandt and Fletcher, 1982; Rucker et al, 1983; Hubbel et al, 1985; Jeavons et al, 1987; Lamers et al, 1989; Archer et al, 1993; Roizen, 1994) and the incidence of abnormal X-rays in our study was comparable with that cited by Kilian et al (1987) and Mehrkens et al (1987) (Table 14).

**Table 13.** Incidence of abnormal X-rays in prospective studies and frequency of complications (meta-analysis).

| Author | Age (years) | Unsuspected results (%) | Relevant to anaesthesia (%) |
|---|---|---|---|
| Maigaard et al (1978) | >30 | 0.2 | 0.0 |
| Lamers et al (1989) | >40 | 0.1 | 0.0 |
| Seymour et al (1982) | >65 | – | 0.0 |
| Törnebrandt and Fletcher (1982) | 70–94 | 11 | – |
| Jeavons et al (1987) | Adults | 2.2 | 0.8 |
| Perez et al (1995) | Adults | 8.6 | 0.56 |
| Rucker et al (1983) | All | 0.3 | 0.0 |
| Haubek and Gold (1978) | 1–94 | 1.9 | 0.0 |
| Petterson and Janover (1977) | All | – | 0.1 |
| Mendelson et al (1987) | All | – | – |
| Hartung (1990) | All | 2.5 | 0.5 |
| Christian et al | All | 22.6 | 3.8 |
| | | 0.1–22 | 0–3.8 |

Modified from Archer et al (1993).

**Table 14.** Incidence of abnormal laboratory results which were normal on repetition.

| Test type | Unexpected abnormal (%) | Normal repeated (%) |
|---|---|---|
| Haematology | 2.9 (Perez et al, 1995) | 15 |
| Biochemical | | 27 |
| Glucose | 2.2 | |
| Gamma-glutamyl transferase (GGT) | 3.2 | |
| Overall | 30–35 (Altemeyer et al, 1984; Kilian et al, 1987; Mehrkens et al, 1987)<br>18 (Lutz et al, 1983)<br>4.3 (McKee and Scott, 1987) | |

From these data it may be concluded that from the 0.1–22% of unexpected abnormal X-ray results observed in the investigated age groups, only a small fraction had a significant influence on the course of anaesthesia, while none was related to complications.

The evaluation of data collected in our prospective study shows the incidence of abnormal X-ray results to be greater in the older patients and, although this was associated with a greater number of complications, these could not be directly correlated with the abnormal X-ray results.

## Laboratory tests

Results reported by Perez et al (1995) indicate that in 2.9% of cases unexpected abnormal findings were detected by haematology tests. Unexpected abnormal biochemical tests had a frequency of 5.6% in their study, with abnormal glucose levels in 2.2% and abnormal GGT in 3.2% of patients. When tests were repeated, 15 out of the total number of 108 abnormal results, and 27 out of 53 abnormal biochemical tests, were within the normal range. Kaplan et al (1985) stated that there was no indication for 60% of the laboratory tests performed in their study. Altemeyer et al (1984), Kilian et al

(1987) and Mehrkens et al (1987) noted abnormal results for laboratory tests in 30–35% and Lutz et al (1983) in 18% of patients, while McKee and Scott (1987) reported abnormal results in only 4.3% of cases.

## ABNORMAL TESTS AND COMPLICATIONS

Although at first glance the intraoperative rates of complications reported by various authors (Lutz et al, 1983; Duncan and Cohen, 1987; Mantha et al, 1994; Mangano, 1995) seem to be at variance, in an analysis of the rates reported for all age groups this difference is greatly diminished: 17% in our study; Lutz et al (1983), 15.6%; List et al (1985), Mehrkens et al (1987) and Hartung (1990), between 16% and 20%. After consideration of all age groups, the haemodynamic complication rate of >80% reported by List et al (1985) and Mehrkens et al (1987) was 53.8% in our study. List et al (1985) found a correlation between pre-operative cardiovascular abnormalities and complications depending on whether the patients were classified as American Society of Anesthesiology (ASA) class III or IV.

One of the reasons for the conflicting results may be the difference in opinion held by various investigators as to what is relevant to anaesthesia. In our study, only major haemodynamic and/or cardiorespiratory complications were recorded and correlated with the results of the pre-operative evaluation.

A further reason may be seen in the fact that in the course of a study certain incidents and events are likely to occur with greater or lesser frequency than outside a study period where complications may also be observed less often. The results of a recent retrospective investigation (Altemeyer et al, 1984) we performed for 2542 patients showed fewer abnormal results in a comparable patient population than observations made in our prospective study (44% compared with 59%).

In patients with an abnormal medical history and physical examination, the ECG was abnormal in only 15% compared with 56% in the prospective study. The same applies to X-rays (8.5% versus 65%) and laboratory tests (5–10% versus 41%).

The representation of ASA groups varied within the two studies in that there were 87% ASA class I+II patients in the retrospective study (study 1) compared with 62% in the prospective study (study 2), 10% ASA class III patients in study 1 and 31% in study 2, and 2% ASA class IV patients in study 1 and 7% in study 2.

Unfortunately, in the retrospective investigation no distinction was made between observations which were relevant to either anaesthesia or outcome and between those of no relevance to either factor. Furthermore, no differentiation could be made between an abnormal and a normal history and the physical examination.

It may therefore be concluded that data obtained by prospective studies are of greater validity than those collected by retrospective or other investigations and that only the former data should serve as the basis for any recommendations.

## COSTS

Vogt and Henson (1997) have concluded from results obtained in 383 patients that 72% of pre-operative laboratory tests ordered by surgeons were not indicated. Had these tests not been performed 'the hospital could generate $80 000 in variable and semifixed cost savings by eliminating these unindicated tests'. Archer et al (1993) stated on the basis of their meta-analysis that by omitting chest X-rays if history and examination are normal 23 US dollars per case could be saved. Roizen (1988) quoted Blue Cross–Blue Shields estimates showing that, out of >30 billion dollars spent on pre-operative testing in North America, 60% could be saved if tests were only ordered when indicated from the history and examination. Kaplan et al (1985) calculated that their institution could save >147,000 US dollars/year if unnecessary tests were omitted. The costs calculated for the small set of examinations performed in our retrospective study in addition to those of the routine medical history and physical examination averaged 115 German marks per patient plus 75 German marks for additional tests required in patients with a positive history and examination.

Should the surgeon request an examination to be performed by a consultant in internal medicine, an amount of 215 DM needs to be added to cover the costs of a highly sophisticated test programme performed by these specialists.

If a somewhat extended battery of routine laboratory tests and ECGs at a cost of 160 DM per patient were performed in 20 000 patients/year at our department, this would result in a total amount of 3.6 million German marks. However, the performance of only a limited number of tests in ASA class 1 patients ($N=2800$), who constitute 14% of our patient population, would result in savings of approximately 432,000 German marks/year.

The cost–benefit ratio therefore needs to be considered when pre-operative tests are ordered. This is of particular importance in patients classified as ASA class I (and II) on the basis of the medical history and physical examination.

## ANSWERS TO THE INITIAL QUESTIONS

(1) The anaesthesia-related medical history and physical examination are the minimum requirement for the pre-operative evaluation.

(2), (3) An anaesthesia-oriented medical history and physical examination should comprise questions related to organ systems which are most obviously affected by anaesthesia and evaluations of body functions influenced by anaesthesia or which, in turn, exert an influence on the course of anaesthesia and the post-operative period.

(4) The percentage of unknown disturbances or disorders detected by ECG, X-ray and laboratory tests is considerable. However, only those previously unknown ECG abnormalities which can be related to complications can be considered to be of relevance to anaesthesia.

(5) Abnormal results do not always influence the anaesthetic manage-

ment and lead to a deferral of the case. They may, however, be related to complications which require particular attention and monitoring.

(6) It is recommended to recheck abnormal test results if they appear suspicious, because not infrequently they return to normal on repetition.

(7) Abnormal test results are relevant to anaesthesia if they can be related to complications or lead to a change in the management of anaesthesia.

(8) It has been shown that patient conditions can be negatively influenced by too many and unindicated investigations, in particular if these are invasive.

(9) The ratio of the per diem cost of deferring a case to a routine pre-operative ECG and laboratory programme is considerable (approximately 650 DM/120 DM).

## RECOMMENDATIONS

Roizen (1994) states that 'our goal has to be efficient delivery of quality care. Studies of perioperative morbidity over four decades repeatedly show that preoperative patient conditions are significant predictors of post-operative morbidity.' A study at the University of Florida found that pre-anaesthetic evaluations provided information leading to changes in care plans for more than 15% of all healthy patients and for 20% of all patients in general. With respect to the fact that (in the US-by far not in Europe-) 70% of all surgical patients are 'outpatients or "come and stay" patients' they 'cannot be evaluated preoperatively as they were in the 1970s.

What are then the conclusions and recommendations that may be drawn from the findings of our studies and those performed by other groups? The one extreme would be to obtain only a sufficiently pertinent medical history and to carry out an anaesthesia-related physical examination. In the majority of cases this will unmask hidden disorders and diseases. Additional tests, i.e. ECG, X-ray and laboratory tests, should only be ordered if the above-mentioned assessments demonstrate abnormalities which may have implications for the course of anaesthesia and/or post-operative recovery. To be effective, however, these activities have to be performed by an experienced anaesthetist (which may not always be guaranteed). The other extreme would be to order and perform routinely a standard battery of tests, including ECG and chest X-rays as well as haematological and biochemical laboratory tests, in order to avoid the possibility of deferring a case because the required additional tests were not carried out.

### Electrocardiograms

Considering that a significant number of abnormal ECG tracings could not be detected by the medical history and physical examination (Gervais et al, 1990) in the younger age groups, the results of our study suggest that an ECG may be indicated independently of patient age, because 5–10% of abnormal findings relevant to anaesthesia were observed even in the younger age groups. In view of the fact that an ECG with the patient at rest is only of limited value (sensitivity–specificity for CAD) we nevertheless recommend that an ECG be obtained for all adults even in the presence of a normal history and physical examination; Roizen (1994) proposes an ECG only for males 40 years and older as well as for both males and females older than 50 years.

**Chest X-ray** (Maigaard et al, 1978; Mendelson et al, 1987)

Roizen (1994) recommends a chest X-ray in patients older than 65 years, but views it as mandatory in the presence of pulmonary disease and smoking. Based on our results we are in agreement with these suggestions and believe that a chest X-ray should not be indicated in otherwise unremarkable patients.

**Laboratory tests** (Lowe et al, 1987; Turnbull and Buck, 1987; Johnson et al, 1988; Christian et al, 1990; Narr et al, 1991; Davies et al, 1994)

*Haemoglobin and haematocrit*

Roizen (1994) suggests that these tests should be ordered in the case of expected blood loss (a factor frequently underestimated by surgeons), in females below the age of 40 years, in all patients older than 65 years and in those with malignancies, renal diseases, smoking and the use of anticoagulants. These recommendations are supported by the results of our study.

*Prothrombin time, partial thromboplastin time, platelet count (PLT) and Quick-Test* (Eisenberg et al, 1982)

In accordance with Roizen (1994) we propose these tests to be ordered only if bleeding disorders are suspected from the medical history and clinical examination and if elective epidural or spinal blocks are performed; they are, furthermore, indicated in patients with liver disease or when anticoagulants are used.

*Electrolytes*

Sodium and potassium levels were never found to be abnormal in patients with an unremarkable history and a normal examination in our study. Even in patients who demonstrated some pathology, sodium concentrations were abnormal in only 0.5% and potassium levels in 0.8%. We therefore do not recommend ordering these tests routinely, provided that the history and examination are normal and there is no suspicion of medication with diuretics, laxants, steroids or digitalis or diabetes, renal and central nervous system disease medication.

*Blood glucose*

Only one of our patients with a normal history and examination had undetected diabetes. This does not justify ordering blood glucose tests routinely in all patients. In 7.4% of our patients with some pathology abnormal blood glucose levels were identified pre-operatively. Blood glucose tests are thus only indicated in known diabetic patients, in patients with central nervous system diseases or in those under treatment with steroids. These tests may also be indicated in patients older than 65 years.

### *Routine hepatic tests*

A relatively low incidence of abnormal liver tests (except GGT) was recorded (Table 15) in our patients with an otherwise normal history.

Liver tests are thus not indicated in all patients: on the one hand they are relatively unspecific (Strunin, 1978; Roizen, 1994) and may, on the other hand, be abnormal in areas where alcohol is regularly consumed (wine-growing areas). A critical situation might occur in patients with a previously undiagnosed, while asymptomatic developing hepatitis; in these patients anaesthesia and operation may have to be deferred (except in urgent cases) or the management needs to be changed. Suspected hepatitis and exposure to hepatitis are the most relevant indications for liver tests.

**Table 15.** Incidence of abnormal liver tests.

| | History and examination (%) | |
|---|---|---|
| Test | Normal | Abnormal |
| GGT | 4 | 10 |
| Serum glutamate pyruvate transaminase (SGPT) | 1 | 3.7 |
| Serum glutamate oxalate transaminase (SGOT) | 0.8 | 2.9 |
| Total protein (TP) | 0.5 | 0.8 |

## CONCLUSION

The primary goal of pre-operative evaluation is to assess conclusively the patient's pre-operative condition and to diagnose and possibly to treat disturbances and diseases which may be of relevance to the course of anaesthesia, surgery and the post-operative period. On the basis of our prospective data and the analysis of relevant factors we have designed a standardized pre-operative evaluation programme (Table 16).

A pertinent medical history and a physical examination are compulsory in all cases and should preferably be performed in the pre-anaesthetic assessment clinic by an experienced anaesthesiologist assisted by an anaesthesia nurse. A specialist internist or any other consultant should only be called on in cases requiring special consideration.

A set of minimal tests, i.e. ECG and GGT, should be carried out for all patients. This is corroborated by our findings showing the values obtained with these tests to be in the abnormal range in a considerable percentage of patients and thus of relevance to anaesthesia and the post-operative period, while the information was not always apparent from the history and the examination.

**Table 16.** Recommendation of a strategy for pre-operative evaluation including indicated additional electrocardiogram, X-ray and laboratory tests.

| | |
|---|---|
| Routinely | 1. Pertinent medical history (N, 28%)<br>2. Physical examination (N, 41%)<br>3. ECG (AN, 14–41%)<br>4. GGT (AN, 10%)<br>We recommend the routine performance of selected coagulation tests if EDA or spinal anaesthetic (SpA) is planned (bleeding time, PTT thrombopectin time (TPT), factor VIII) |
| Only if indicated | Laboratory<br>Haematocrit (Hct) (AN, 0–3.5%)<br>Blood glucose (AN, 0–6.5%) |
| Based on history and examination | $K^+$ (AN, 0–2%) |

N, normal history and examination; AN, unexpected abnormal test results.

The costs for these investigations are approximately 48.00 German marks per patient. Further laboratory tests such as haematocrit, blood glucose and potassium are only ordered if indicated based on the history and examination at an additional cost of 28 DM, increasing the total cost for the complete set to 76 German marks.

The performance of this small set of tests is justified for at least two reasons. First, the expenses incurred at our hospital even for the more extensive laboratory, ECG and X-ray programme average 123 DM compared with 760 DM for each day of deferred surgery. Second, at least in some European countries the anaesthesiologist is required by law to order basic laboratory tests in all cases where an abnormal result may be expected (i.e. diabetes) if the corresponding pre-existing medication is continued.

Roizen (1994) has discussed this aspect under the heading 'The danger of underordering tests'. He holds underordering responsible for 15% of all problems or operating room delays (even in ASA physical status (PS) class I cases).

A certain minimal pre-operative programme consisting of two sub-programmes therefore needs to be performed, in order to be able to meet

**Table 17.** Recommendations for a stepwise pre-anaesthetic evaluation programme.

| | |
|---|---|
| 1. Anaesthesia-related medical history and physical examination | In all patients |
| 2. ECG | In all patients |
| 3. GGT | In all cases (at least in wine-growing regions) |
| 4. Only if indicated | |
| a. Quick test, partial thromboplastin time, thrombocytes, PLT | Regional anaesthesia<br>Bleeding disorders<br>Medication |
| b Haemoglobin, Hct, K, SGOT–SGPT, alkaline phosphatase, creatinine, blood glucose | If indicated |
| c. Lung function test, chest X-ray | If indicated |
| 5. More specific tests depending on pre-existing disease or medication (Christian et al, 1988, 1990; Dick, 1990; Fleisher and Beattie, 1993; American College of Cardiology–American Heart Association Task Force, 1996) | |

our primary goal while avoiding unindicated invasive diagnostic measures and treatment as well as unjustified costs:

- subprogramme I, required in all elective cases;
- subprogramme II, requested only if additional symptoms are revealed by the history and examination.

In special high-risk patients decisions as to treatment must be made according to the needs of the individual patient.

Recommendations for a pre-anaesthetic evaluation programme are listed in Table 17.

## REFERENCES


Altemeyer KH, Schultz M, Mehrkens HH et al (1984) Pre-operative evaluation of 2500 patients in a pre-anaesthetic assessment clinic. *Anästhesiologie und Intensivmedizin* **25:** 1 (in German).

*American College of Cardiology–American Heart Association Task Force (1996) Guidelines for perioperative cardiovascular evaluation for noncardiac surgery. *Journal of Cardiothoracic and Vascular Surgery* **10:** 540–552.

Archer C, Levy AR & McGregor M (1993) Value of routine preoperative chest x-rays a metaanalysis. *Canadian Journal of Anaesthesia* **40:** 1022–1027.

Callaghan LC, Edwards ND & Reilly CS (1995) Utilisation of the pre-operative ECG. *Anaesthesia* **50:** 488–490.

*Christian KW, Gervais H & Dick W (1988) Pre-operative screening and anaesthetic risk. *Anästhesist* **37:** 694–703 (in German).

Christian KW, Gervais H & Dick W (1990) Pre-operative evaluation: laboratory tests. *Anästhesiologie und Intensivmedizin* **4:** 108–109 (in German).

Davies JM, Pagenkopf D, Todd K et al (1994) Comparison of selection of preoperative laboratory tests: the computer vs the anaesthetist. *Canadian Journal of Anaesthesia* **41:** 1156–1160.

Diamond GA & Forrester JS (1979) Analysis of probability as an aid in the clinical diagnosis of coronary artery disease. *New England Journal of Medicine* **300:** 1350–1358.

Dick WF (1990) The calculation of 'anaesthesiability'. *Anästhesiologie und Intensivmedizin* **31:** 66–67, 150–151 (in German).

*Dick W, Ahnefeld FW, Fricke M et al (1978) The anaesthesia out-patient clinic. *Anästhesist* **27:** 450–458 (in German).

Duncan PG & Cohen MM (1987) Postoperative complications: factors of significance to anaesthetic practice. *Canadian Journal of Anaesthesia* **34:** 12–18.

Eisenberg JU, Clarke JR & Sussman SA (1982) Prothrombin and partial thromboplastin times as preoperative screening tests. *Archives of Surgery* **117:** 48–51.

Feddersen K (1990) Preoperative assessment. *Current Opinion in Anaesthesiology* **3:** 53–56.

Fischer K (1990) Assessment of readiness for anaesthesia—financial aspects. *Anästhesiologie und Intensivmedizin* **5:** 144–146 (in German).

Fleisher LA & Beattie C (1993) Current practice in the preoperative evaluation of patients undergoing major vascular surgery: a survey of cardiovascular anesthesiologists. *Journal of Cardiothoracic and Vascular Anesthesia* **7:** 650–654.

Gervais H, Christian KW & Dick W (1990) Pre-operative evaluation: ECG. *Anästhesiologie und Intensivmedizin* **4:** 103–104 (in German).

Gold BS, Young ML, Kinman JL et al (1992) The utility of preoperative electrocardiograms in the ambulatory surgical patient. *Archives of Internal Medicine* **152:** 301–305.

Goldman L (1987) The art and science of perioperative consultation. *Journal of General and Internal Medicine* **2:** 284–285.

Hartung HJ (1990) Pre-operative investigation: X-ray and lung function tests. *Anästhesiologie und Intensivmedizin* **4:** 105–107 (in German).

Haubek A & Gold G (1978) Praeoperative rontgenuntersogelse af thorax, indikation og konsegvens. *Ugeskrift for Laeger* **140:** 766–768.

Hubbel FA, Greenfield S, Tyler J et al (1985) The impact of routine admission chest X-ray films on patient care. *New England Journal of Medicine* **312:** 209–213.

Hyman AI (1990) Preoperative assessment of the patient with cardiovasular disease. *Current Opinion in Anaesthesiology* **3:** 35–39.

Jeavons SJ, Siddle KJ, Mitchell C & O'Hare PM (1987) Evaluation of chest x-ray. *Australasian Radiology* **31:** 256–259.

Johnson H, Knee-ioli S, Butler T et al (1988) Are routine preoperative laboratory screening tests necessary to evaluate ambulatory surgical patients? *Surgery* **104:** 639–645.

*Kaplan EB, Sheiner LB, Boeckmann AJ et al (1985) The usefulness of preoperative laboratory screening. *Journal of the American Medical Association* **253:** 3576–3581.

Kellerer AM (1991) Risk assessment. *Medizinische Klinik* **8(6):** 109–111 (editorial) (in German).

Kilian J, Pauly P & Altemeyer KH (1987) Experiences with a standardized pre-operative evaluation programme. In *Proceedings of the Central European Congress of Anaesthesiology*, p 826 (in German).

Lamers RJS, Van Engelshoven JMA & Pfaff A (1989) Nogmals, de routinematige preoperatieve thoraxfoto. *Nederlands Tijdschrift voor Geneeskunde* **133:** 2288–2291.

*Lee A, Lum ME, Perry M et al (1993) Risk of unanticipated intraoperative events in patients assessed at preanaesthetic clinic. *Canadian Journal of Anaesthesia* **44:** 946–954.

List WF, Kröll W & Filzwieser G (1985) Peri-operative risk of severely ill surgical patients. *Anästhesist* **34:** 612–618 (in German).

Lowe RA, Wood AB, Burney RE & Mackenzie JR (1987) Rational ordering of serum electrolytes: development of clinical criteria. *Annals of Emergency Medicine* **16:** 260–269.

Lutz H, Oswald PM & Bender HJ (1983) Is a routine pre-operative evaluation programme justified? *Anästhesiologische und Intenzivmedizinische Notfallmedizin* **18:** 153–155 (in German).

Maigaard S, Ekljaer P & Stefansson TU (1978) Value of routine preoperative radiographic examination of the thorax and ECG. *Ugeskrift for Laeger* **140:** 769–771 (abstract).

*Mangano DT (1995) Preoperative risk assessment: many studies, few solutions. *Anesthesiology* **83:** 897–901.

*Mantha S, Roizen MF, Barnard J et al (1994) Relative effectiveness of four preoperative tests for predicting adverse cardiac outcomes after vascular surgery: a metaanalyis. *Anesthesia and Analagesia* **79:** 422–433.

McKee RF & Scott EM (1987) The value of routine preoperative investigations. *Annals of the Royal College of Surgeons of England* **69:** 160–162.

Mehrkens HH, Schultz M & Walther FG (1987) On the importance of additional tests for the preoperative evaluation. *Proceedings of the Central European Congress of Anaesthesiology*, p 832 (in German).

Mendelson DS, Khilnani N, Wagner LP & Rabinowitz JG (1987) Preoperative chest radiography: value as a baseline examination for comparison. *Radiology* **165:** 341–343.

Narr BJ, Hansen TR & Warren MA (1991) Preoperative laboratory screening in healthy Mayo patients: cost effective elimination of tests and unchanged outcomes. *Mayo Clinic Proceedings* **66:** 155–159.

Oswald PM, Hartung HJ & Feldmann U (1985) Prognostic significance of a pre-operative risk check list. *Anästhesist* **34:** 508–512 (in German).

Paraskos JA (1992) Who needs a preoperative electrocardiogram? *Archives of Internal Medicine* **152:** 261–263.

Perez A, Planell J, Bacardaz C et al (1995) Value of routine preoperative tests: a multicenter study in four general hospitals. *British Journal of Anaesthesia* **74:** 250–256.

Petterson SR & Janover ML (1977) Is the routine preoperative film of value? *Applied Radiology* **6:** 70.

Roizen MF (1988) The compelling rationale for less preoperative testing. *Canadian Journal of Anaesthesia* **35:** 214–218 (editorial).

*Roizen MF (1994) Preoperative evaluation. IARS Review Course Lectures Suppl. *Anaesth Analg* 78–85.

Rucker L, Frye EB & Staten MA (1983) Usefulness of screening chest roentgenograms in preoperative patients. *Journal of the American Medical Association* **250:** 3209–3211.

Seymour DG, Pringl R & Shaw JW (1982) The role of the routine preoperative chest X-ray in the elderly general surgical patient. *Postgraduate Medical Journal* **58:** 741–745.

Strunin L (1978) Preoperative assessment of the patient with liver dysfunction. *British Journal of Anaesthesia* **50:** 25–28.

Törnebrandt K & Fletcher R (1982) Preoperative chest X-rays in elderly patients. *Anaesthesia* **37:** 901–902.

Turnbull JM & Buck C (1987) The value of preoperative screening investigations in otherwise healthy individuals. *Archives of Internal Medicine* **147:** 1101–1105.

*Vogt AW & Henson LC(1997) Unindicated preoperative testing: ASA physical status and financial implications. *Journal of Clinical Anaesthesia* **9:** 437–441.

4

# Pre-operative cardiac evaluation before non-cardiac surgery

LEE A. FLEISHER MD

Associate Professor of Anesthesiology and Critical Care Medicine, and Joint Appointment in Medicine (Cardiology) and Health Policy and Management
*The Johns Hopkins Hospital, 600 N. Wolfe Street Carnegie 442, Baltimore, Maryland 21287, USA*

Several recent guidelines have been published to codify the pre-operative evaluation of the cardiac patient undergoing non-cardiac surgery. Considering the lack of any randomized clinical trials in this area, they have incorporated information from both prospective cohort studies and the experience from the general care of the cardiac patient. The decision to perform testing is based on the clinical risk factors, exercise tolerance and surgical procedure. Testing should not be performed unless the results will actually change practice. Among the interventions advocated to reduce peri-operative risk, the decision to perform coronary revascularization before non-cardiac surgery must include issues related to local rates of morbidity and mortality for each of the procedures and potential long-term benefits.

**Key words:** pre-operative evaluation; cardiac evaluation; testing; revascularization; guidelines.

The optimal pre-operative cardiac evaluation of high-risk patients undergoing non-cardiac surgery has been an area of great interest to anaesthesiologists, internists and surgeons for over 20 years. In the current era of cost containment, the rational use of expensive testing has taken on an even greater importance. Two groups have recently published guidelines on pre-operative cardiac testing, but with different approaches and purposes. The American College of Cardiology–American Heart Association (AHA) has published Guidelines on Perioperative Cardiovascular Evaluation for Noncardiac Surgery and has attempted to define the optimal peri-operative management for the high-risk patient based on the evidence and expert opinion (Eagle et al, 1996). In contrast, the American College of Physicians (Palda and Detsky, 1997) has also recently published guidelines, the purpose of which is to delineate an evidence-based approach to pre-operative risk stratification. Therefore, the latter document focuses less on the information needed to manage the patient optimally than on the strength

*Baillière's Clinical Anaesthesiology*—
Vol. 12, No. 3, September 1998
ISBN 0–7020–2536–4
0950–3501/98/030373 + 18 $12.00/00

of the evidence for risk assessment and diagnostic testing. This review will discuss these two guidelines from the perspective of the practising anaesthesiologist's desire to care optimally for the high-risk patient.

## PATHOPHYSIOLOGICAL FOUNDATIONS FOR PRE-OPERATIVE CARDIAC EVALUATION

A basic tenet in pre-operative evaluation is that information regarding the extent and stability of disease will affect patient management and lead to improved outcome. In the case of cardiovascular disease, the pre-operative evaluation attempts to define the extent of coronary artery disease (CAD) and the left ventricular function. Numerous studies have attempted to identify those factors which lead to peri-operative cardiac morbidity. Virtually all identify the presence of peri-operative myocardial ischaemia as the strongest predictor of risk (Mangano et al, 1990; Raby et al, 1992; Fleisher et al, 1995a). Therefore, much of the pre-operative evaluation has focused on identifying the 'ischaemic potential' and individual response to ischaemia.

Once the probability of developing myocardial ischaemia or significant CAD is assessed on clinical grounds, the decision regarding the value of further diagnostic test depends on how the information will be used. Delineation of risk may determine the need for invasive monitoring or post-operative intensive care resources. For example, in a patient undergoing aortic aneurysm resection, a randomized trial demonstrated no difference in outcome between use of a central venous pressure or pulmonary artery catheter in patients without redistribution on dipyridamole thallium imaging (Isaacson et al, 1990). In patients who are identified as having extensive CAD, coronary revascularization can be considered (see later in chapter). Finally, intensive resources may not be available in all locations and further defining extent of disease may lead to a referral to a higher-acuity hospital.

Several authors have suggested that extensive evaluation is no longer necessary in an era of low cardiac morbidity (Seeger et al, 1994; D'Angelo et al, 1997). They argue that improvements in intra- and post-operative care obviates the need for an extensive evaluation. However, the studies that support the low rate of morbidity are frequently from academic institutions with intensive resource utilization. Using claims data, we have found that 30 day mortality after major vascular surgery is over 8% in an unselected cohort of individuals over age 65 years (Fleisher et al, 1997). Therefore, it is important to document low morbidity and mortality prior to abandoning the practice of pre-operative evaluation.

## CARDIAC RISK INDICES

Since the original manuscript by Goldman et al (1977) describing a cardiac risk index, multiple investigators have validated various clinical risk indices for their ability to predict peri-operative cardiac complications. The Goldman Cardiac Risk Index originally defined nine factors, each of which was given a weight or number of points (Table 1). The total number of points ascribed to a given individual was calculated and the patient was placed into one of four classes, each of which was associated with an increasing rate of peri-operative cardiac morbidity. The cardiac risk index has been validated in large populations of diverse types of non-cardiac surgery but does not appear as robust in selected populations of patients undergoing major vascular surgery. Detsky et al (1986) modified the cardiac risk index, adding factors such as major vascular surgery and angina (Table 2). The patients were placed into one of three classes based on the total number of points. The American College of Physicians guidelines, written by Palda and Detsky (1997), defined the Detsky modification of the cardiac risk index as the clinical approach which has the strongest evidence for support. Importantly, the American Society of Anesthesiologists physical status classification performs almost as well as either cardiac risk index. From the anaesthesiologist's perspective, a classification of risk does not provide sufficient information to modify peri-operative care appropriately; rather, the anaesthesiologist needs information regarding the potential for developing myocardial ischaemia and the ventricular reserve of the patient. Therefore, such indices may be useful in defining baseline risk but are not useful for refining peri-operative management.

**Table 1.** Computation of the cardiac risk index.

| Criteria* | Multivariate discriminant function coefficient | Points |
|---|---|---|
| I. History | | |
| (a) Age >70 years | 0.191 | 5 |
| (b) MI in previous 6 months | 0.384 | 10 |
| II. Physical examination | | |
| (a) $S_3$ gallop or JVD | 0.451 | 11 |
| (b) Important VAS | 0.119 | 3 |
| III. Electrocardiogram | | |
| (a) Rhythm other than sinus or PACs on last pre-operative ECG | 0.283 | 7 |
| (b) >5 PVCs/min documented at any time before operation | 0.278 | 7 |
| IV. General status | | |
| $PO_2$ <60 or $PCO_2$ >50 mmHg, K <3.0 or $HCO_3$ <20 mEq/l, BUN >50 or Cr >3.0 mg/dl, abnormal SGOT, signs of chronic liver disease or patient bedridden from non-cardiac causes | 0.132 | 3 |
| V. Operation | | |
| (a) Intraperitoneal, intrathoracic or aortic operation | 0.123 | 3 |
| (b) Emergency operation | 0.167 | 4 |
| Total possible points | | 53 |

* MI, myocardial infarction; JVD, jugular-vein distension; VAS, valvular aortic stenosis; PACs, premature atrial contractions; ECG, electrocardiogram; PVCs, premature ventricular contractions; $PO_2$, partial pressure of oxygen; $PCO_2$, partial pressure of carbon dioxide; K, potassium; $HCO_3$, bicarbonate; BUN, blood urea nitrogen; Cr, creatinine; SGOT, serum glutamic oxalacetic transminase. Reproduced from Goldman et al (1977, *New England Journal of Medicine* **297:** 845–850) with permission.

**Table 2.** Modified cardiac risk index by Detsky et al (1986).

| Variables | Points |
|---|---|
| Angina | 20 |
| Class IV | 20 |
| Class III | 10 |
| Unstable angina <3 months | 10 |
| Suspected critical aortic stenosis | 20 |
| MI | |
| <6 months | 10 |
| >6 months | 5 |
| Alveolar pulmonary oedema | |
| <1 week | 10 |
| Ever | 5 |
| Emergency surgery | 10 |
| Sinus plus atrial premature beats or rhythm other than sinus on pre-operative ECG | 5 |
| >5 PVCs at any time before surgery | 5 |
| Poor general medical status | 5 |
| Age >70 years | 5 |

Reproduced from Detsky et al (1986, *Journal of General and Internal Medicine* **1:** 211–219) with permission.

## CLINICAL RISK FACTORS

A thorough history should focus on cardiovascular risk factors and symptoms or signs of unstable cardiac disease states such as myocardial ischaemia, congestive heart failure, valvular heart disease and significant cardiac arrhythmias.

In patients with symptomatic coronary disease, the pre-operative evaluation may lead to the recognition of a change in the frequency or pattern of anginal symptoms. Symptoms of cardiovascular disease should be carefully determined, especially characteristics of chest pain, if present. Certain populations of patients, for example the elderly, women or diabetics, may present with more atypical features. One study found that chest pain was a presenting feature of angina pectoris in only approximately 40% of individuals >85 years of age. The presence of unstable angina has been associated with a high peri-operative risk of MI (Shah et al, 1990a). The peri-operative period is associated with a hypercoagulable state and surges in endogenous catecholamines, both of which may exacerbate the underlying process in unstable angina, increasing the risk of acute infarction (Tuman et al, 1991). The pre-operative evaluation can impact on both short- and long-term health of a patient by instituting treatment of unstable angina.

The patient with stable angina represents a continuum from mild angina with extreme exertion to dyspnoea with angina after walking up a few stairs. The patient who only manifests angina after strenuous exercise does not demonstrate signs of left ventricular dysfunction and would not be a candidate for changes in management. In contrast, a patient with dyspnoea on mild exertion would be at high risk for developing peri-operative ventricular dysfunction, myocardial ischaemia and possible MI. These patients have an extremely high probability of having extensive CAD and additional monitoring or cardiovascular testing should be contemplated, depending on the surgical procedure and institutional factors.

In virtually all studies, the presence of active congestive heart failure pre-operatively has been associated with an increased incidence of peri-operative cardiac morbidity (Goldman et al, 1977; Detsky et al, 1986). Stabilization of ventricular function and treatment for pulmonary congestion are prudent prior to elective surgery. Also, it is important to determine the aetiology of the left heart failure. Congestive symptoms may be due to non-ischaemic cardiomyopathy or mitral or aortic valvular insufficiency and/or stenosis. Because the type of peri-operative monitoring and treatments would be different, clarifying the cause of cardiac congestion is important.

Patients with a prior MI have CAD, although a small group of patients may sustain an MI from a non-atherosclerotic mechanism. Traditionally, risk assessment for non-cardiac surgery was based on the time interval between the MI and surgery. Multiple studies have demonstrated an increased incidence of re-infarction if the MI was within 6 months of surgery (Tarhan et al, 1972; Rao et al, 1983; Shah et al, 1990b) (Table 1). With improvements in peri-operative care, this difference has decreased.

However, the importance of the intervening time interval may no longer be valid in the current era of thrombolytics, angioplasty and risk stratification after an acute MI. Although many patients with an MI may continue to have myocardium at risk for subsequent ischaemia and infarction, other patients may have their critical coronary stenosis either totally occluded or widely patent. For example, the use of percutaneous transluminal coronary angioplasty (PTCA) is associated with a reduced incidence of death or re-infarction within 6 months. Therefore, patients should be evaluated from the perspective of their risk for ongoing ischaemia. The AHA–American College of Cardiology Task Force on Perioperative Evaluation of the Cardiac Patient Undergoing Noncardiac Surgery (Table 3) has advocated the use of an MI <30 days as the group at highest risk, while, after that period, risk stratification is based on the presentation of disease and exercise tolerance (Eagle et al, 1996).

## Patients at risk for coronary artery disease

For those patients without overt symptoms or history, the probability of CAD varies with the type and number of atherosclerotic risk factors present. Peripheral arterial disease has been shown to be associated with CAD in multiple studies. Hertzer et al (1984) studied 1000 consecutive patients scheduled for major vascular surgery and found that approximately 60% of patients had at least one coronary artery with a critical stenosis.

Diabetes mellitus is common in the elderly and represents a disease that impacts on multiple organ systems. Complications of diabetes mellitus are frequently the cause of urgent or emergency surgery, especially in the elderly. Diabetes accelerates the progression of atherosclerosis, which can be frequently silent in nature. Diabetics have a higher probability of CAD than non-diabetics do. There is a high incidence of both silent MI and

**Table 3.** Cardiac risk* stratification for non-cardiac surgical procedures.

| | |
|---|---|
| High | Reported cardiac risk often >5%<br>• Emergent major operations, particularly in the elderly<br>• Aortic and other major vascular<br>• Peripheral vascular<br>• Expected prolonged surgical procedures associated with large fluid shifts and/or blood loss |
| Intermediate | Reported cardiac risk generally <5%<br>• Carotid endarterectomy<br>• Head and neck<br>• Intraperitoneal and intrathoracic<br>• Orthopaedic<br>• Prostate |
| Low† | Reported cardiac risk generally <1%<br>• Endoscopic procedures<br>• Superficial procedure<br>• Cataract<br>• Breast |

* Combined incidence of cardiac death and non-fatal MI.
† Do not generally require further pre-operative cardiac testing.
Reproduced from Eagle et al (1996, *Circulation* **93:** 1278–1317) with permission.

myocardial ischaemia (Kannel and Abbott, 1984). Eagle et al (1989) demonstrated that diabetes is an independent risk factor for peri-operative cardiac morbidity. In attempting to determine the degree of this increased probability, the length of the disease and other associated end-organ dysfunction should be taken into account. Autonomic neuropathy has recently been found to be the best predictor of silent CAD (Acharya et al, 1991). Because these patients are at very high risk for silent MI, the electrocardiogram should be obtained to examine for the presence of Q waves.

Hypertension has also been associated with an increased incidence of silent myocardial ischaemia and infarction (Kannel and Abbott, 1984). Those hypertensive patients with left ventricular hypertrophy and who are undergoing non-cardiac surgery are at a higher peri-operative risk than non-hypertensive patients (Hollenberg et al, 1992). Investigators have suggested that the presence of a strain pattern on ECG suggests a chronic ischaemic state (Pringle et al, 1989). Therefore, these patients should also be considered to have an increased probability of CAD and developing cardiovascular morbidity.

There is a great deal of debate regarding a trigger to delay or cancel a surgical procedure in a patient with poorly or untreated hypertension. Although Goldman and Caldera (1979) suggested that a case should be delayed if the diastolic pressure is greater than 110 mmHg, they demonstrated no major morbidity in this small cohort of individuals in their study. In the absence of end-organ changes, such as renal insufficiency or left ventricular hypertrophy with strain, it would seem appropriate to proceed with surgery. In contrast, a patient with a markedly elevated blood pressure and the new onset of a headache should have surgery delayed for further treatment.

Several other risk factors have been used to suggest an increased probability of CAD. These include the atherosclerotic processes associated with tobacco use and hypercholesterolaemia. Although these risk factors increase the probability of developing CAD, they have not been shown to increase peri-operative risk. When attempting to determine the overall probability of disease, the number and severity of the risk factors are important.

## IMPORTANCE OF SURGICAL PROCEDURE

The surgical procedure influences the extent of the pre-operative evaluation required by determining the potential range of changes in peri-operative management. For example, a pulmonary artery catheter or trans-oesophageal echocardiography may be appropriate for a patient undergoing major abdominal or vascular surgery, but would not be considered appropriate for ambulatory surgery. Similarly, coronary revascularization may be beneficial for procedures associated with a high incidence of morbidity and mortality, but not those associated with a low incidence, as described below. There are few hard data to define the surgery-specific incidence of complications. It is known that peripheral procedures, such as those included in a study of ambulatory surgery completed at the Mayo Clinic, are associated with an extremely low incidence of morbidity and mortality (Warner et al, 1993). Similarly, major vascular procedures are associated with among the highest incidence of complications, with a similar incidence documented for infrainguinal and aortic surgery (Krupski et al, 1992). Eagle et al (1997) published data on the incidence of peri-operative MI and mortality by procedure for patients enrolled in the Coronary Artery Surgery Study (CASS). They determined the overall risk of peri-operative morbidity in patients with known CAD on medical treatment and the potential reduced rate of peri-operative morbidity in those patients who had a prior coronary artery bypass grafting (CABG). High-risk procedures include major vascular, abdominal, thoracic and orthopaedic surgery. The AHA–American College of Cardiology Guidelines defined three tiers of surgical stress, which are shown in Table 3 (Eagle et al, 1996).

## IMPORTANCE OF EXERCISE TOLERANCE

Exercise tolerance is one of the most important determinants of peri-operative risk and the need for invasive monitoring (McPhail et al, 1988). An excellent exercise tolerance, even in patients with stable angina, suggests that the myocardium can be stressed without becoming dysfunctional. If a patient can walk a mile without becoming short of breath, then the probability of extensive CAD is small. Alternatively, if patients become dyspnoeic associated with chest pain during minimal exertion, then the probability of extensive CAD is high. A greater degree of CAD has been associated with a higher peri-operative risk (Fleisher et al, 1995b). Additionally, these patients are at risk for developing hypotension with ischaemia, and therefore may benefit from more extensive monitoring or coronary revascularization. Exercise tolerance can be assessed with formal treadmill testing or with a questionnaire which assessed activities of daily living (Table 4) (Eagle et al, 1996).

**Table 4.** Estimated energy requirement for various activities*.

| | | | |
|---|---|---|---|
| 1 MET | Can you take care of yourself? | 4 METs | Climb a flight of stairs or walk up a hill? |
| | Eat, dress, or use the toilet? | | Walk on level ground at 4 mph or 6.4 km/h? |
| | Walk indoors around the house? | | Run a short distance? |
| | Walk a block or two on level ground at 2–3 mph or 3.2–4.8 km/h? | | Do heavy work around the house like scrubbing floors or lifting or moving heavy furniture? |
| | Do light work around the house like dusting or washing dishes? | | Participate in moderate recreational activities such as golf, bowling, dancing, doubles tennis, or throwing a baseball or football? |
| | | >10 METs | Participate in strenuous sports like swimming, singles tennis, football, basketball, or skiing? |

MET indicates metabolic equivalent.
* Adapted from the Duke Activity Status Index and AHA Exercise Standards.
Reproduced from Eagle et al (1996, *Circulation* **93:** 1278–1317) with permission.

## APPROACH TO THE PATIENT

The algorithm to determine the need for testing proposed by the American College of Cardiology–AHA Task Force is based on the available evidence and expert opinion and integrates clinical history, surgery-specific risk and exercise tolerance (Figure 1). First, the clinician must evaluate the urgency of the surgery and the appropriateness of a formal pre-operative assessment. Next, determine whether the patient has undergone a previous revascularization procedure or coronary evaluation. Those patients with unstable coronary syndromes should be identified, and appropriate treatment instituted. Finally, the decision to undergo further testing depends on the interaction of the clinical risk factors (Table 5), surgery-specific risk and functional capacity. For patients at intermediate clinical risk, both the exercise tolerance and the extent of the surgery are taken into account with regard to the need for further testing. Importantly, no pre-operative cardio-

**Figure 1 (see page 373).** The AHA–American College of Cardiology Task Force on Perioperative Evaluation of Cardiac Patients Undergoing Noncardiac Surgery has proposed an algorithm for decisions regarding the need for further evaluation. This represents one of multiple algorithms proposed in the literature. It is based on expert opinion and incorporates six steps. First, the clinician must evaluate the urgency of the surgery and the appropriateness of a formal pre-operative assessment. Next, he or she must determine whether the patients has had a previous revascularization procedure or coronary evaluation. Those patients with unstable coronary syndromes should be identified, and appropriate treatment should be instituted. The decision to have further testing depends on the interaction of the clinical risk factors, surgery-specific risk, and functional capacity. CHF, congestive heart failure. Adapted from Eagle et al (1996, *Circulation* **93:** 1278–1317).

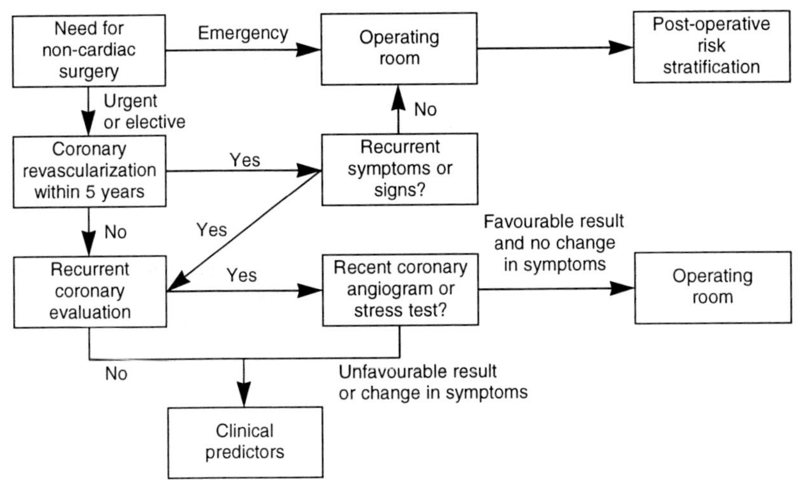
Need for non-cardiac surgery
Emergency
Operating room
Post-operative risk stratification
Urgent or elective
No
Coronary revascularization within 5 years
Yes
Recurrent symptoms or signs?
No
Yes
Favourable result and no change in symptoms
Recurrent coronary evaluation
Yes
Recent coronary angiogram or stress test?
Operating room
No
Unfavourable result or change in symptoms
Clinical predictors

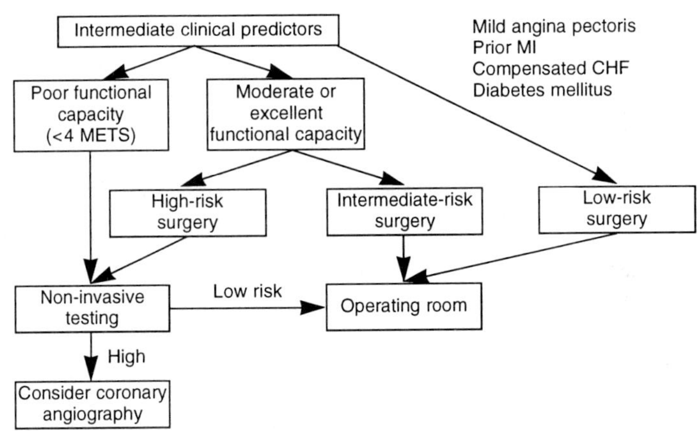
Intermediate clinical predictors
Mild angina pectoris
Prior MI
Compensated CHF
Diabetes mellitus
Poor functional capacity (<4 METS)
Moderate or excellent functional capacity
High-risk surgery
Intermediate-risk surgery
Low-risk surgery
Non-invasive testing
Low risk
Operating room
High
Consider coronary angiography

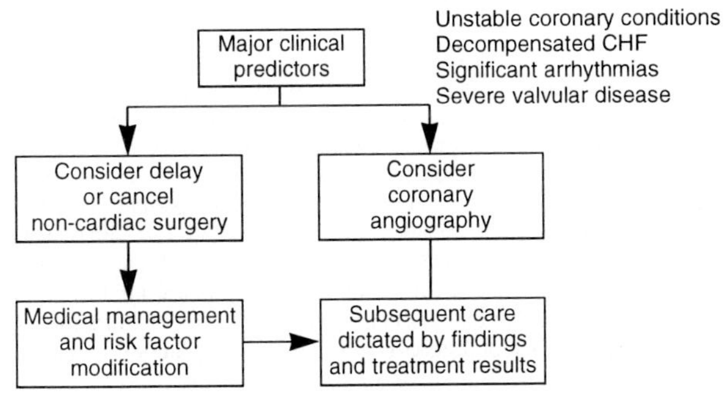
Major clinical predictors
Unstable coronary conditions
Decompensated CHF
Significant arrhythmias
Severe valvular disease
Consider delay or cancel non-cardiac surgery
Consider coronary angiography
Medical management and risk factor modification
Subsequent care dictated by findings and treatment results

**Table 5.** Clinical predictors of increased peri-operative cardiovascular risk (myocardial infarction, congestive heart failure, death).

Major

Unstable coronary syndromes

- Recent MI* with evidence of important ischaemic risk by clinical symptoms or non-invasive study
- Unstable or severe† angina (Canadian class III or IV)‡

Decompensated congestive heart failure

Significant arrhythmias

- High-grade atrioventricular block
- Symptomatic ventricular arrhythmias in the presence of underlying heart disease
- Supraventricular arrhythmias with uncontrolled ventricular rate

Severe valvular disease

Intermediate

Mild angina pectoris (Canadian class I or II)

Prior MI by history or pathological Q waves

Compensated or prior congestive heart failure

Diabetes mellitus

Minor

Advanced age

Abnormal ECG (left ventricular hypertrophy, left bundle branch block, ST–T abnormalities)

Rhythm other than sinus (e.g. atrial fibrillation)

Low functional capacity (e.g. inability to climb one flight of stairs with a bag of groccries)

History of stroke

Uncontrolled systemic hypertension

* The American College of Cardiology National Database Library defines recent MI as greater than 7 days but less than or equal to 1 month (30 days).

† May include 'stable' angina in patients who are unusually sedentary.

‡ Campeau (1976).

Reproduced from Eagle et al (1996, *Circulation* **93:** 1278–1317) with permission.

---

**Figure 2 (see page 375).** The American College of Physicians Guidelines for assessing and managing the peri-operative risk from CAD associated with major non-cardiac surgery. The commentary in italics represents the strength of evidence to support each decision process in the algorithm. An evidence-based analysis of the literature accompanied the algorithm in a paper by Palda and Detsky (1997). Initially, patients are assessed using the Detsky modification of the cardiac risk index to determine whether they are class I (low risk) or class II or III (high risk). If they are class I, clinical predictors such as those identified by Eagle are collected to determine whether they represent low or high clinical risk. Only those patients with several clinical predictors are then determined to be at intermediate peri-operative risk. Those patients with an intermediate risk and undergoing vascular surgery should be considered for non-invasive imaging with dipyridamole thallium imaging or dobutamine stress echocardiography. No further testing is suggested in those patients undergoing non-vascular surgery. If the non-invasive testing is positive or the patient is at high clinical Detsky risk, then it is important to determine the nature of the risk. If the risk is largely due to ischaemic heart disease, then it is important to determine whether the patient would be eligible for coronary revascularization based on AHA Guidelines independent of non-cardiac surgery. If the risk is due to non-ischaemic origins then the ideal choice is to optimize and reassess. Finally, if it is due to largely non-modifiable factors then either cancelling the case or modifying the non-cardiac surgery should be considered. DTI = dipyridamole thallium imaging; DSE = dobutamine stress echocardiography. Reproduced from Palda and Detsky (1997, *Annals of Internal Medicine* **127:** 313–328) with permission.

vascular testing should be performed if the results will not change perioperative management.

The American College of Physicians Guidelines attempt to apply the evidence-based approach (Figure 2) (Palda and Detsky, 1997). The initial decision point is the assessment of risk using the Detsky modification of the cardiac risk index (Detsky et al, 1986). If the patient is class II or III, they are considered high risk. If they are class I, the presence of other clinical factors according to work by Eagle et al (1989) or Vanzetto et al (1996) is used to stratify risk further. Those with multiple markers for cardiovascular disease according to these risk indices and undergoing major vascular

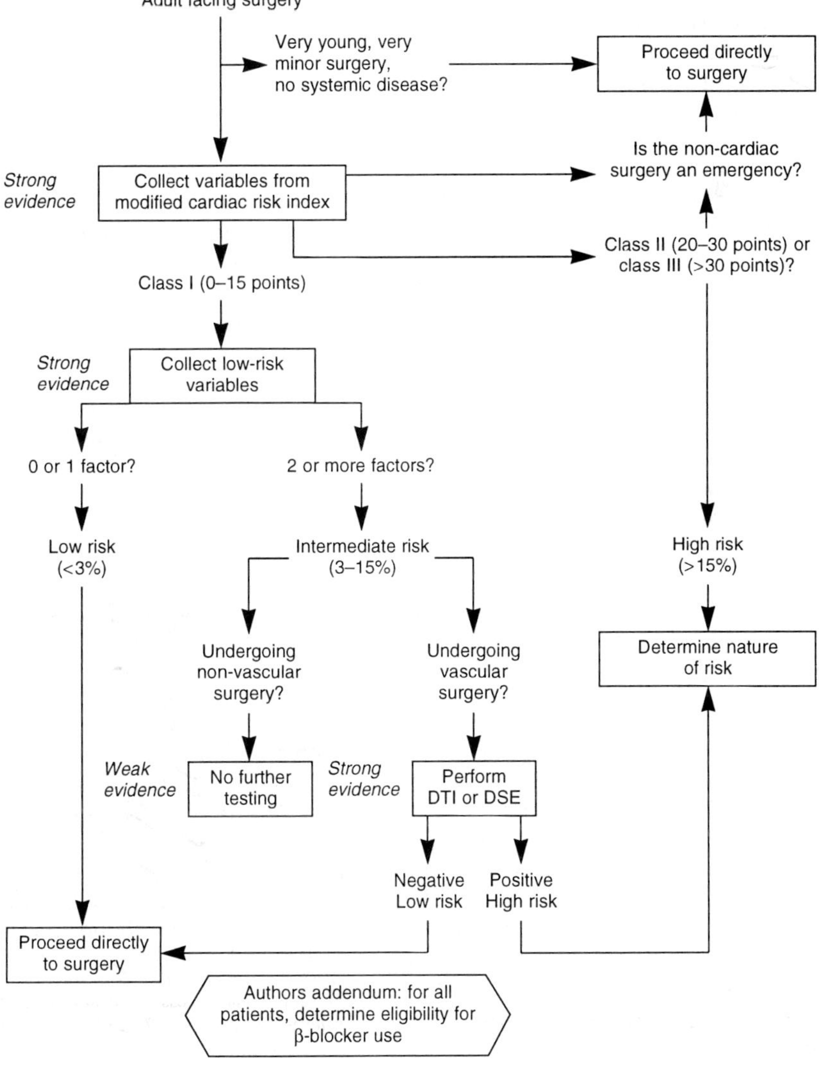

surgery are considered appropriate for further diagnostic testing by either dipyridamole imaging or dobutamine stress echocardiography. The guidelines suggest that there is insufficient evidence to recommend diagnostic testing for non-vascular surgery patients.

## CORONARY REVASCULARIZATION (see Chapter 7 for details)

Before cardiovascular testing is performed, it is important to determine whether the results will impact on peri-operative management. Among the various interventions, several investigators have proposed coronary revascularization before non-cardiac surgery as a means of reducing peri-operative risk. There are no randomized trials to address this issue, and such a trial would require a very large sample size and have multiple confounding issues (Cohen et al, 1995). However, there are several large cohort studies which suggest that, in patients who survive CABG, the risk of subsequent non-cardiac surgery is low (Huber et al, 1992; Eagle et al, 1997). While there are few data to support the notion of coronary revascularization solely for the purpose of improving peri-operative outcome, it is true that for specific patient subsets long-term survival may be enhanced by revascularization. Rihal et al (1992) utilized the CASS database and found that CABG significantly improved survival in those patients with both peripheral vascular disease and triple-vessel coronary disease, especially the group with depressed ventricular function.

The value of PTCA is less well established. In several series, a low incidence of cardiovascular complications was observed in patients undergoing 'prophylactic' PTCA before vascular surgery, but it is difficult to determine the expected complication rate in a comparison group with single- or double-vessel disease (Allen et al, 1991; Huber et al, 1992). For those peri-operative MIs that result from plaque rupture and coronary thrombosis in non-critical lesions, as seen in the ambulatory setting, single-vessel PTCA of more critical stenoses will theoretically have minimal benefit. Ellis et al (1996) studied 21 patients who had coronary angiography before major vascular surgery and sustained a peri-operative cardiac event. None of the MIs occurred in areas distal to a critical stenosis, while approximately one-third occurred distal to non-critical stenoses (Ellis et al, 1996). Therefore, the current evidence does not support the use of PTCA beyond established indications for non-operative patients.

An alternative approach to determining the optimal strategy for medical care in the absence of clinical trials is construction of a decision analysis. Two decision analyses have been published on the issue of cardiovascular testing before major vascular surgery (Figure 3) (Fleisher et al, 1994; Mason et al, 1995). Both assumed that patients with significant CAD would undergo CABG prior to non-cardiac surgery. Both models found that the optimal decision was sensitive to local morbidity and mortality rates within the clinically observed range. These models suggest that pre-operative testing for the purpose of coronary revascularization is not the optimal strategy if peri-operative morbidity and mortality are low.

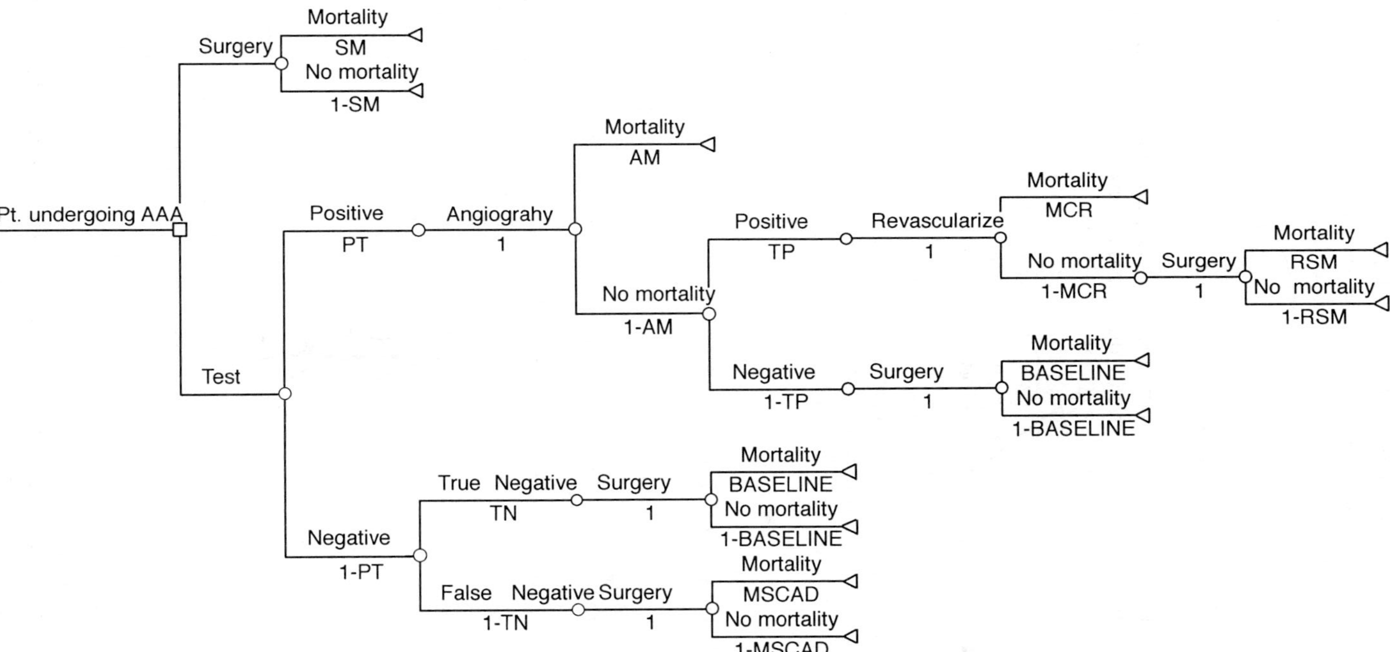


**Figure 3.** A decision algorithm evaluating the decision between vascular surgery alone or coronary artery revascularization before vascular surgery. There are currently no randomized trials to address the optimal strategy. By outlining the multiple decision points at which a patient can sustain mortality by choosing to undergo coronary revascularization first, the optimal strategy for pre-operative evaluation can be demonstrated. Specifically, variation in mortalities at each decision point can change the optimal strategy. Adapted from Fleisher et al (1994, *Anesthesia and Analgesia* **79:** 661–669).

Importantly, the primary cost (in both dollars and morbidity) of pre-operative testing and revascularization is the revascularization procedure itself. Therefore, the indications for revascularization, and thus the frequency of its use, have a significant impact on the model. Second, potential long-term benefits of coronary revascularization in this population were not included in the analysis, potentially biasing against the revascularization arm. If long-term survival is included in the models, then coronary revascularization may lead to improved overall outcome and be a cost-effective intervention. However, a patient's age should be included in the equation. For example, an 80 year old diabetic patient with significant co-morbid diseases may gain few additional life years and may actually have a decrease in the quality of their final years by undergoing coronary revascularization. In contrast, a 55 year old man with an abdominal aortic aneurysm who is found to have occult left main disease would have a substantial increase in both the length and the quality of his life from pre-operative cardiovascular testing and coronary revascularization. Therefore, identification of appropriate patients with diffuse disease or a significant left main stenosis amenable to surgery with an acceptable risk should undergo CABG before non-cardiac surgery. In this instance, the procedure is justified based on long-term benefit and performing it before non-cardiac surgery reduces the risk of a fatal or non-fatal peri-operative MI.

## CHOICE OF DIAGNOSTIC TEST

There are multiple non-invasive diagnostic tests which have been proposed to evaluate the extend of CAD before non-cardiac surgery. The exercise electrocardiogram has been the traditional method of evaluating individuals for the presence of CAD. It represents the least invasive and most cost-effective method of detecting ischaemia, with a reasonable sensitivity (68–81%) and specificity (66–77%) for identifying CAD (Detrano et al, 1989). The goal of the test is to provoke ischaemia through exercise, by causing an increase in myocardial oxygen demand relative to myocardial oxygen supply. Electrocardiographic signs of myocardial ischaemia and clinical signs of left ventricular dysfunction are considered positive. However, as outlined above, patients with a good exercise tolerance will rarely benefit from further testing.

A significant number of high-risk patients either are unable to exercise or have contraindications to exercise. In surgical patients, this phenomenon is most evident in those patients with claudication or an abdominal aortic aneurysm undergoing vascular surgery, both of which have a high rate of peri-operative cardiac morbidity. Therefore, pharmacological stress testing has become popular, particularly as a pre-operative test in vascular surgery patients.

Pharmacological stress tests for the detection of CAD can be divided into two categories: (1) those that result in coronary artery vasodilation such as dipyridamole and (2) those that increase myocardial oxygen demand such as dobutamine. The coronary artery vasodilators work by producing differential flows in normal coronary arteries when compared with those with a stenosis. Several authors have shown that the presence of a redistribution defect on dipyridamole thallium imaging in patients undergoing peripheral vascular surgery is predictive of post-operative cardiac events (Boucher et al, 1985; Cutler and Leppo, 1987; Eagle et al, 1987; Lette et al, 1992). This work has been extended to include patients undergoing non-vascular surgery (Fleisher et al, 1995b). In order to increase the predictive value of the test, several strategies have been suggested. Lung uptake, left ventricular cavity dilation and redistribution defect size have all been shown to be predictive of subsequent morbidity. Fleisher et al (1995b) demonstrated that the delineation of 'low' and 'high' risk thallium scans markedly improved the test's predictive value. They demonstrated that only patients with 'high' risk thallium scans were at increased risk for peri-operative morbidity and long-term mortality.

The ambulatory ECG (AECG or Holter) provides a means of continuously monitoring the ECG for significant ST segment changes during the pre-operative period. Raby et al (1989) demonstrated that the presence of silent ischaemia is a strong predictor of outcome, while its absence was associated with a good outcome in 99% of patients. Other investigators have demonstrated the value of silent AECG monitoring, although the negative predictive values have not been as high as originally reported (Fleisher et al, 1995b). Fleisher et al (1995b) demonstrated a similar predictive value of dipyridamole thallium imaging and AECG monitoring; however, the quantity of silent ischaemia could not be used to identify those patients at greatest risk who might benefit from further testing and coronary revascularization.

Stress echocardiography has received attention as a pre-operative test. The appearance of new or worsened regional wall motion abnormalities is considered a positive test. These represent areas at risk for myocardial ischaemia. The advantage of this test is that it is a dynamic assessment of ventricular function. Dobutamine echocardiography has also been studied and found to have among the best positive and negative predictive value (Poldermans et al, 1993). Poldermans et al (1995) demonstrated that the group at greatest risk were those who demonstrated regional wall motion abnormalities at low heart rates.

Several groups have recently published meta-analyses of pre-operative diagnostic tests. Mantha et al (1994) demonstrated good predictive values of AECG monitoring, radionuclide angiography, dipyridamole thallium imaging and dobutamine stress echocardiography. Shaw et al (1996) also demonstrated good predictive values of dipyridamole thallium imaging and dobutamine stress echocardiography. Both studies demonstrated the superior predictive value of dobutamine stress echocardiography; however, there was significant overlap of the confidence intervals with other tests. However, the most important determinant with respect to the choice of pre-operative testing is the expertise at the local institution. The decision to perform further invasive testing and management should be based on the principles outlined above, i.e. the ability of the intervention to affect both short- and long-term health.

## SUMMARY

Two recent guidelines have attempted to distil the available knowledge and evidence regarding pre-operative cardiovascular evaluation and testing. Testing is of value in high-risk patients undergoing major vascular surgery. The decision to perform further evaluation in other situations depends on the interactions of patients and surgery-specific factors, as well as exercise capacity.

## REFERENCES

Acharya DU, Shekhar YC, Aggarwal A & Anand IS (1991) Lack of pain during myocardial infarction in diabetics—is autonomic dysfunction responsible? *American Journal of Cardiology* **68:** 793–796.

Allen J, Helling T & Hartzler G (1991) Operative procedures not involving the heart after percutaneous transluminal coronary angioplasty. *Surgery, Gynecology and Obstetrics* **173:** 285–288.

D'Angelo AJ, Puppala D, Farber A et al (1997) Is preoperative cardiac evaluation for abdominal aortic aneurysm repair necessary? *Journal of Vascular Surgery* **25(1):** 152–156.

Boucher CA, Brewster DC, Darling RC et al (1985) Determination of cardiac risk by dipyridamole-thallium imaging before peripheral vascular surgery. *New England Journal of Medicine* **312:** 389–394.

Campeau L (1976) Grading of angina pectoris. *Circulation* **54:** 522–523.

Cohen MC, McKenna C, Lewis SM & Muller JE (1995) Requirements for controlled clinical trials of preoperative cardiovascular risk reduction. *Controlled Clinical Trials* **16(2):** 89–95.

Cutler BS & Leppo JA (1987) Dipyridamole thallium 201 scintigraphy to detect coronary artery disease before abdominal aortic surgery. *Journal of Vascular Surgery* **5(1):** 91–100.

Detrano R, Gianrossi R, Mulvihill D et al (1989) Exercise-induced ST segment depression in the diagnosis of multivessel coronary disease: a meta analysis. *Journal of the American College of Cardiology* **14:** 1501–1508.

Detsky A, Abrams H, McLaughlin J et al (1986) Predicting cardiac complications in patients undergoing non-cardiac surgery. *Journal of General and Internal Medicine* **1:** 211–219.

Eagle KA, Singer DE, Brewster DC et al (1987) Dipyridamole-thallium scanning in patients undergoing vascular surgery. Optimizing preoperative evaluation of cardiac risk. *Journal of the American Medical Association* **257(16):** 2185–2189.

*Eagle KA, Coley CM, Newell JB et al (1989) Combining clinical and thallium data optimizes preoperative assessment of cardiac risk before major vascular surgery. *Annals of Internal Medicine* **110:** 859–866.

*Eagle K, Brundage B, Chaitman B et al (1996) Guidelines for perioperative cardiovascular evaluation of the noncardiac surgery. A report of the American Heart Association/American College of Cardiology Task Force on Assessment of Diagnostic and Therapeutic Cardiovascular Procedures. *Circulation* **93:** 1278–1317.

*Eagle KA, Rihal CS, Mickel MC et al (1997) Cardiac risk of noncardiac surgery: influence of coronary disease and type of surgery in 3368 operations. CASS Investigators and University of Michigan Heart Care Program. Coronary Artery Surgery Study. *Circulation* **96(6):** 1882–1887.

Ellis SG, Hertzer NR, Young JR & Brener S (1996) Angiographic correlates of cardiac death and myocardial infarction complicating major nonthoracic vascular surgery. *American Journal of Cardiology* **77(12):** 1126–1128.

*Fleisher LA, Skolnick ED, Holroyd KJ & Lehmann HP (1994) Coronary artery revascularization before abdominal aortic aneurysm surgery: a decision analytic approach. *Anesthesia and Analgesia* **79:** 661–669.

Fleisher LA, Eagle KA, Shaffer T & Anderson G (1997) Mortality after major vascular surgery: analysis of the Medicare database. *Anesthesia and Analgesia* **84:** SCA43 (abstract).

Fleisher LA, Nelson AH & Rosenbaum SH (1995a) Postoperative myocardial ischemia: etiology of cardiac morbidity or manifestation of underlying disease. *Journal of Clinical Anesthesia* **7:** 97–102.

Fleisher LA, Rosenbaum SH, Nelson AH et al (1995b) Preoperative dipyridamole thallium imaging and Holter monitoring as a predictor of perioperative cardiac events and long term outcome. *Anesthesiology* **83:** 906–917.

Goldman L & Caldera DL (1979) Risks of general anesthesia and elective operation in the hypertensive patient. *Anesthesiology* **50:** 285–292.

*Goldman L, Caldera DL, Nussbaum SR et al (1977) Multifactorial index of cardiac risk in noncardiac surgical procedures. *New England Journal of Medicine* **297:** 845–850.

Hertzer NR, Bevan EG, Young JR et al (1984) Coronary artery disease in peripheral vascular patients: a classification of 1000 coronary angiograms and results of surgical management. *Annals of Surgery* **199:** 223–233.

Hollenberg M, Mangano DT, Browner WS et al (1992) Predictors of postoperative myocardial ischemia in patients undergoing noncardiac surgery. The Study of Perioperative Ischemia Research. *Journal of the American Medical Association* **268:** 205–209.

Huber KC, Evans MA, Bresnahan JF et al (1992) Outcome of noncardiac operations in patients with severe coronary artery disease successfully treated preoperatively with coronary angioplasty. *Mayo Clinic Proceedings* **67:** 15–21.

Isaacson IJ, Lowdon JD, Berry AJ et al (1990) The value of pulmonary artery and central venous monitoring in patients undergoing abdominal aortic reconstructive surgery: a comparative study of two selected, randomized groups. *Journal of Vascular Surgery* **12(6):** 754–760.

Kannel W & Abbott R (1984) Incidence and prognosis of unrecognized myocardial infarction: an update on the Framingham Study. *New England Journal of Medicine* **311:** 1144–1147.

Krupski WC, Layug EL, Reilly LM et al (1992) Comparison of cardiac morbidity between aortic and infrainguinal operations. Study of Perioperative Ischemia (SPI) Research Group. *Journal of Vascular Surgery* **15(2):** 354–363.

Lette J, Waters D, Cerino M et al (1992) Preoperative coronary artery disease risk stratification based on dipyridamole imaging and a simple three-step, three-segment model for patients undergoing noncardiac vascular surgery or major general surgery. *American Journal of Cardiology* **69:** 1553–1558.

McPhail N, Calvin JE, Shariatmadar A et al (1988) The use of preoperative exercise testing to predict cardiac complications after arterial reconstruction. *Journal of Vascular Surgery* **7(1):** 60–68.

*Mangano DT, Browner WS, Hollenberg M et al (1990) Association of perioperative myocardial ischemia with cardiac morbidity and mortality in men undergoing noncardiac surgery. *New England Journal of Medicine* **323:** 1781–1788.

Mantha S, Roizen MF, Barnard J et al (1994) Relative effectiveness of four preoperative tests for predicting adverse cardiac outcomes after vascular surgery: a meta-analysis. *Anesthesia and Analgesia* **79(3):** 422–433.

Mason JJ, Owens DK, Harris RA et al (1995) The role of coronary angiography and coronary revascularization before noncardiac surgery. *Journal of the American Medical Association* **273:** 1919–1925.

Palda VA & Detsky AS (1997) Perioperative assessment and management of risk from coronary artery disease. *Annals of Internal Medicine* **127:** 313–328.

Poldermans D, Fioretti PM, Forster T et al (1993) Dobutamine stress echocardiography for assessment of perioperative cardiac risk in patients undergoing major vascular surgery. *Circulation* **87(5):** 1506–1512.

*Poldermans D, Arnese M, Fioretti PM et al (1995) Improved cardiac risk stratification in major vascular surgery with dobutamine–atropine stress echocardiography. *Journal of the American College of Cardiology* **26(3):** 648–653.

Pringle SD, MacFarlane PW, McKillop JH et al (1989) Pathophysiologic assessment of left ventricular hypertrophy and strain in asymptomatic patients with essential hypertension. *Journal of the American College of Cardiology* **13:** 1377–1381.

Raby KE, Goldman L, Creager MA et al (1989) Correlation between perioperative ischemia and major cardiac events after peripheral vascular surgery. *New England Journal of Medicine* **321:** 1296–1300.

Raby KE, Barry J, Creager MA et al (1992) Detection and significance of intraoperative and postoperative myocardial ischemia in peripheral vascular surgery. *Journal of the American Medical Association* **268:** 222–227.

Rao TK, Jacobs KH & El-Etr AA (1983) Reinfarction following anesthesia in patients with myocardial infarction. *Anesthesiology* **59:** 499–505.

Rihal C, Gersh B, Whisnant J et al (1992) Influence of coronary heart disease on morbidity and mortality after carotid endarterectomy: a population-based study in Olmsted County, Minnesota (1970–1988). *Journal of the American College of Cardiology* **19:** 1254–1260.

Seeger JM, Rosenthal GR, Self SB et al (1994) Does routine stress–thallium cardiac scanning reduce postoperative cardiac complications? *Annals of Surgery* **219(6):** 654–651.

Shah KB, Kleinman BS, Rao T et al (1990a) Angina and other risk factors in patients with cardiac diseases undergoing noncardiac operations. *Anesthesia and Analgesia* **70:** 240–247.

Shah KB, Kleinman BS, Sami H et al (1990b) Reevaluation of perioperative myocardial infarction in patients with prior myocardial infarction undergoing noncardiac operations. *Anesthesia and Analgesia* **71:** 231–235.

Shaw LJ, Eagle KA, Gersh BJ & Miller DD (1996) Meta-analysis of intravenous dipyridamole-thallium-201 imaging (1985 to 1994) and dobutamine echocardiography (1991 to 1994) for risk stratification before vascular surgery. *Journal of the American College of Cardiology* **27(4):** 787–798.

Tarhan S, Moffitt EA, Taylor WF & Giuliani ER (1972) Myocardial infarction after general anesthesia. *Journal of the American Medical Association* **220:** 1451–1454.

Tuman KJ, McCarthy RJ, March RJ et al (1991) Effects of epidural anesthesia and analgesia on coagulation and outcome after major vascular surgery. *Anesthesia and Analgesia* **73(6):** 696–704.

Vanzetto G, Machecourt J, Blendea D et al (1996) Additive value of thallium single-photon emission computed tomography myocardial imaging for prediction of perioperative events in clinically selected high cardiac risk patients having abdominal aortic surgery. *American Journal of Cardiology* **77(2):** 143–148.

Warner MA, Shields SE & Chute CG (1993) Major morbidity and mortality within 1 month of ambulatory surgery and anesthesia. *Journal of the American Medical Association* **270(12):** 1437–1441.

# 5

# The pulmonary risk patient

ANDREAS ZOLLINGER MD

Consultant and Senior Lecturer

THOMAS PASCH MD

Professor and Chairman

*Institute of Anaesthesiology, University Hospital Zürich, Rämistrasse 100, CH-8091 Zürich, Switzerland*

Chronic pulmonary diseases are among the leading causes of death, and pulmonary complications are frequent causes of peri-operative morbidity and mortality in thoracic and in non-thoracic surgery. Pre-operative risk assessment is important to prevent peri-operative complications. It is the aim of this chapter to review recent reports on peri-operative pulmonary risk factors and to discuss controversial aspects. Patients at risk in non-thoracic surgery are best identified by a detailed history, careful clinical examination and overall co-morbidity scoring systems. Pulmonary function tests, however, do not predict peri-operative complications and therefore should not be used alone to decide on the patient's operability. Also, conventional, so-called prohibitive lung function parameters should no longer be used to deny a potentially curative resection of lung tissue. Alternatively, more significant parameters need to be identified. Because evidence-based data are not available, an interdisciplinary approach to specific problems of severely compromised or co-morbid patients is mandatory.

**Key words:** pulmonary disease; peri-operative complications; risk; lung function test; lung volume reduction; lung volume measurement; surgery; anaesthesia.

Chronic pulmonary diseases, mainly chronic obstructive pulmonary disease (COPD) and lung emphysema, are among the leading causes of death in all industrialized countries. The incidence of chronic lung disease rises further with the increasing mean age of the population. Furthermore, bronchogenic carcinoma, usually caused by smoking, is one of the most common causes of cancer death in these countries. Smoking, on the other hand, is associated not only with severe lung disease but often with cardio-vascular diseases. Therefore, in clinical practice, the anaesthesiologist is frequently faced with a combination of severe respiratory and cardio-vascular impairment. Pulmonary complications are among the major causes


ISBN 0-7020-2536-4
0950-3501/98/030391 + 13 $12.00/00

of peri-operative morbidity and mortality in thoracic as well as in non-thoracic surgery (Lawrence et al, 1996; McCulloch et al, 1997; Rady et al, 1997; Mitchell et al, 1998; Weiner et al, 1998).

In order to prevent peri-operative respiratory complications, it is generally accepted that peri-operative risk assessment is an important tool that allows the morbidity and mortality associated with both thoracic and non-thoracic surgery to be reduced. Therefore, pre-operative recognition of pulmonary risk factors and, if possible, adequate pre-treatment of patients at risk, are mandatory. Many aspects of pre-operative pulmonary risk assessment and of anaesthesia for the patient with severe pulmonary disease have been reviewed recently (Melendez and Fischer, 1997; Domino, 1998). It is the aim of this chapter to review recent reports on peri-operative pulmonary risk factors and complications and to discuss the controversies about the pulmonary risk factors for non-thoracic surgery as well as the role of the so-called prohibitive lung function for pulmonary resection.

## PRE-OPERATIVE ASSESSMENT OF PULMONARY RISK FACTORS

In 1961, Mittman stated 'The ideal assessment of operative risk would identify every patient who could safely tolerate surgery. This ideal is probably unattainable . . .' (Mittman, 1961). Unfortunately, this is still true today. Several studies in large numbers of patients have analysed the correlation between pulmonary risk factors and peri-operative risk. However, the specific risk for the individual patient cannot be predicted reliably. Too many variables, which are potentially interrelated, are involved (i.e. the underlying disease, co-morbid conditions, pre-existing medication, drug, alcohol and nicotine addiction, age, sex, type and duration of surgery and anaesthesia etc.). Furthermore, the impact of rapidly evolving anaesthetic techniques, including monitoring devices, alternative surgical methods and intensive care concepts, on morbidity and mortality is unknown. One might assume that they all contribute to a better quality of patient management. Hence, results of older studies on peri-operative risk may no longer be valid (Kearney et al, 1994), and reports published more than 15 years ago (Olsen et al, 1975; Miller et al, 1981) must be interpreted with great caution (Cerfolio et al, 1996). This is particularly true if so-called 'prohibitive' lung function parameters which were derived from these reports (e.g. 'cut-off' value for predicted post-operative forced expiratory volume in 1 second (ppo$FEV_1$) at 0.8 l (Olsen et al, 1975)) are used to determine the feasibility of tumour resection or lung volume reduction surgery (LVRS) in patients with lung cancer or severe end-stage pulmonary emphysema. A number of recent studies indicate that this approach of pre-operative pulmonary risk assessment, although still widely used, may be inappropriate. Finally, when assessing the operative risk, one should also consider the risk of denying a potentially curative operation (Table 1), which still remains the only therapeutic option in many cases.

**Table 1.** Risk assessment.

| | |
|---|---|
| Considering the risk | • to do something<br>• to refrain from doing something<br>• to do nothing (not to do anything) |

Specific questions have to be answered at the time of pre-operative risk assessment of each individual patient. 'Operability', 'resectability' and 'risk of anaesthesia' are frequently addressed by both doctors and patients. Unfortunately, these terms are not unequivocally defined in the literature. The definitions used in this chapter are given in Table 2. Furthermore, the type and site of surgery have to be specified. In a study by Wong et al (1995), for example, abdominal incision was identified as an important independent risk factor for post-operative pulmonary complications in patients with severe COPD. However, most earlier data have been obtained in patients scheduled for thoracic procedures, mainly lung resection. Therefore, the results and conclusions of these studies should not be directly applied to non-thoracic procedures or to cardiovascular operations. Finally, the definition of a 'pulmonary complication' is different between studies and may also differ in clinical use. Therefore, results have to be interpreted, compared and translated into clinical practice with great caution.

**Table 2.** Terminology: definitions.

| Term | Application | Definition |
|---|---|---|
| Operability | All types of surgery | The cardiopulmonary reserves are sufficient to survive the planned operation |
| Resectability | Lung resection | Technical feasibility of lung (tumour) resection<br>The planned lung resection will be tolerated without chronic disability |
| Anaesthetic risk | All types of surgery | Peri-operative risk related to anaesthetic methods |

## Evaluation of lung function

The clinical evaluation of the patient (detailed history and physical examination) is the most important part of routine pre-operative assessment of pulmonary function. This examination should include assessment of dyspnoea in patients with severe respiratory distress using an appropriate score (Task Group on Screening for Respiratory Disease in Occupational Settings, 1982; Mahler et al, 1984; Gift and Narsavage, 1998). Chest radiographs and computed tomographic scans, if available, have to be studied carefully. Usual pulmonary function tests include measurement of lung volumes, assessment of maximum breathing capacity and peak expiratory flow rate (American Thoracic Society, 1987; Quanjer et al, 1993) and measurement of carbon monoxide diffusion capacity (DLCO) (Cotes et al, 1993). Exercise testing to evaluate the cardiopulmonary reserve of a patient can be performed by stair climbing (Van Nostrand et al, 1968; Bolton et al, 1987), measurement of 6 or 12 minutes walking distance (McGavin et al, 1976; Bernstein et al, 1994), treadmill walking (Beaumont et al, 1985) or cycle spiroergometry with assessment of maximum oxygen consumption ($\dot{V}O_2$ max) (Bechard and Wetstein, 1987). Arterial blood-gas analysis is the standard method to assess the gas exchange of the spontaneously breathing patient at room air or with supplemental oxygen. Techniques to predict post-operative pulmonary function include simple mathematical calculations (based on a loss of 5.26% for each segment resected (Juhl and Frost, 1975)), measurement of oxygen uptake in different parts of the lung using bronchospirometry (Neuhaus and Cherniak, 1968) and so-called split lung function testing using radionuclide scintigraphy (Boysen et al, 1977). The latter technique allows the estimation of the perfusion of the lung for which resection is planned. When non-significant ventilation–perfusion mismatching is assumed, ppo$FEV_1$ can be calculated and maximum exercise data can be predicted accurately by this method (Larsen et al, 1997a). Pre-operative right heart catheterization with the measurement of pulmonary artery pressure and the calculation of pulmonary vascular resistance (PVR) may be indicated in selected cases only. However, the indications are controversial and data are not conclusive (Reilly et al, 1993). Alternatively, right heart function and pulmonary artery pressure can be estimated less invasively using transthoracic echocardiography. However, in patients with severe lung hyperinflation due to pulmonary emphysema, this method is not suitable in clinical practice because the quality of echo images is usually poor. Transoesophageal echocardiography, on the other hand, may be troublesome in patients with severe dyspnoea.

## ARE THE PULMONARY RISK FACTORS IN PATIENTS FOR NON-THORACIC SURGERY REALLY KNOWN?

In clinical practice, patients with severe pulmonary impairment frequently present for general, non-thoracic surgery. Pre-operative identification of individual risk factors that predict peri-operative pulmonary complications would be of great value. A number of recent studies have addressed this specific topic. However, intra- and post-operative pulmonary complications have been defined differently by different authors, and studies have been performed in different patient populations scheduled for different surgical interventions. It is obvious that not all complications are equivalent and therefore cannot be compared in one analysis (Wong et al, 1995). Hence, it is difficult, if not impossible, to compare the results of these different studies and to draw any conclusions.

The methods and results of studies published within the last 3 years are summarized in Table 3. None of these studies could identify a pre-operative pulmonary factor, i.e. one or more lung function parameters obtained by spirometry, as an independent risk factor for post-operative pulmonary complications. On the contrary, more complex scoring systems which

**Table 3.** Post-operative pulmonary complications following elective non-thoracic surgery: methods and important results of recent studies.

| Reference | Methods | Results | |
|---|---|---|---|
| Bluman et al (1998) | • 'Non-cardiac elective surgery'<br>• Prospective cohort<br>• Effect of smoking behaviour<br>• Smoking history self-report | PPC current smokers<br>past smokers<br>never smokers | 22.0%<br>12.8%<br>4.9% |
| Mitchell et al (1998) | • 'General elective surgery'<br>• Prospective survey<br>• Patient age >40 years<br>• Multivariate analysis | PPC<br>+ post-operative nasogastric intubation<br>pre-operative sputum production<br>longer anaesthesia duration | 11% |
| McCulloch et al (1997) | • 'Head and neck surgery'<br>• Retrospective review<br>• Uni- and multivariate analysis | PPC<br>+ smoking history<br>peri-operative antibiotic choice<br>(pre-operative weight loss) | 15% |
| Brooks-Brunn (1997) | • 'Abdominal surgery'<br>• Prospective<br>• Multivariate, logistic regression | PPC<br>+ independent:<br>age ≥60 years<br>impaired cognitive function<br>smoking history past 8 weeks<br>body mass index ≥27<br>cancer history<br>incision site upper abdominal | – |
| Lawrence et al (1996) | • 'Elective abdominal surgery'<br>• Retrospective (case control)<br>• Multivariate analysis | PPC<br>+ independent:<br>Charlson co-morbidity index<br>Goldman cardiac risk index<br>abnormal chest radiograph<br>abnormal lung examination<br>– lung spirometry | 5% |
| Hall et al (1996) | • 'Abdominal surgery'<br>• Prospective<br>• Logistic regression analysis | 'Respiratory insufficiency'<br>+ ASA class >2<br>presence of chronic bronchitis | 3% |
| Wong et al (1995) | • 'Non-cardiothoracic surgery'<br>• Patients with severe COPD: $FEV_1 \leq 1.2$ l or $FEV_1/FVC < 75\%$<br>• Multivariate analysis | PPC<br>+ Shapiro score ≥5<br>ASA class ≥4<br>– pre-operative pulmonary factors | 37% |

ASA, American Society of Anesthesiologists; $FEV_1$, forced expiratory volume in 1 second; FVC, forced vital capacity; PPC, post-operative pulmonary complications; +, positive predictors for post-operative pulmonary complications; –, not predictive for post-operative pulmonary complications.

assess overall co-morbidity, such as the ASA physical status grade (ASA classification), the Goldman cardiac risk index, the Charlson co-morbidity index or the Shapiro score, were the best predictors of complications (Table 3). This may be explained, partly, by the high rate of co-morbidity in patients with severe respiratory impairment. On the other hand, post-operative cardiac dysfunction may often be accompanied or followed by respiratory compromise, and vice versa. In fact, Lawrence et al (1996) reported both cardiac and respiratory complications in 33% of all cases. Hence, the isolated identification of pulmonary or cardiovascular risk factors alone may be impossible and, in many cases, even inappropriate. Combined prediction of both types of complications rather than a single complication appears to meet the clinical requirements of pre-operative risk assessment better in these patients. However, simple physical and radiological lung examination (Hall et al, 1996; Lawrence et al, 1996) and detailed assessment of the patient's history, primarily of his or her smoking history, of sputum production and of the presence of chronic bronchitic symptoms (Brooks-Brunn, 1997; McCulloch et al, 1997; Bluman et al, 1998; Mitchell et al, 1998), appear to be good predictors for complications (Table 3). This type of clinical risk assessment is cost effective and may reduce the patient's stress associated with most of the more technical examinations. Furthermore, while performing a careful physical examination, it is the anaesthetist's chance to be directly involved in the pre-operative evaluation and risk assessment of his patient and hence to improve his own impact on peri-operative patient management.

In summary, a number of different independent pulmonary risk factors and potentially interrelated variables have been indentified. However, for the individual patient, the specific risk of post-operative pulmonary complications is not easy to define. Detailed assessment of the patient's history and careful clinical examination are of utmost importance to identify patients at increased pulmonary risk. Overall co-morbidity, as assessed by multifactorial scoring systems, like the ASA physical status classification, appears to be directly associated with post-operative pulmonary complications. However, pulmonary function tests do not predict peri-operative complications and therefore should not be used alone to decide on the operability of a patient for non-thoracic surgery.

## PROHIBITIVE LUNG FUNCTION FOR PULMONARY RESECTION: FACT OR FICTION?

In patients evaluated for lung resection the detailed pre-operative assessment of pulmonary function and of pulmonary risk factors is regarded as a matter of course. It is traditionally the pneumologist who assesses the resectability in patients with malignant or chronic inflammatory lung diseases. On the basis of the lung function and other diagnostic tools as summarized above, he or she identifies patients who might not tolerate a planned lung resection. Therefore, the definition of a clear-cut so-called 'prohibitive lung function' appears to be mandatory. From the anaesthesiological point of view, however, this issue needs to be observed critically.

### Pulmonary resection for lung tumour and infection

Gaensler et al (1954) retrospectively analysed the course of patients after lung resection for tuberculosis. These authors were the first to report on a correlation between vital capacity, maximum breathing capacity and post-operative outcome (Gaensler et al, 1954). Since then, however, an increasing number of parameters, either as single values or as combined, more complex indices, have been used to predict post-operative lung function and post-operative morbidity and mortality. The commonly cited and clinically used parameters are summarized in Table 4. Unfortunately, however, it is currently more confusing than ever in the past. These traditional cut-off values have been questioned by many authors. Cerfolio et al (1996) recently stated 'The previous concept of a minimal ppo$FEV_1$ of 0.8 l may no longer be applicable with new anesthetic and critical care techniques. We were unable to identify any specific preoperative pulmonary function test as a predictor of postoperative morbidity.' Kearney et al (1994) concluded 'Pulmonary resection should not be denied on the basis of traditionally cited preoperative pulmonary variables, and a prediction of postoperative pulmonary function by a technique of simple calculation may be useful to identify patients at risk for medical complications.' Are there any valuable alternatives to these traditional values?

On the basis of work by Zibrak et al (1990), Melendez and Fischer (1997) recently presented a summary of the predictive value (discriminative power) of various pre-operative tests: each test was analysed with respect to its sensitivity and specificity to predict 'complication'. According to this list, the authors defined three predictive value groups (Table 5) and suggested the use of a flow decision chart for the pre-operative evaluation of patients for lung resection. However, this concept gives rise to some concerns. First are the different tests aimed at prediction of different outcome criteria, i.e. 'medical complication', 'pulmonary complication' and 'death'. For example, spirometry and the PPP (Pierce et al, 1994) were analysed as predictors of death, and $VO_2$ max at 40 W as well as the PRQ (Barrera and Melendez, 1996) were analysed as predictors of pulmonary

**Table 4.** Commonly used cut-off values associated with a prohibitive lung function for pulmonary resection in patients with bronchogenic carcinoma.

| Parameter | Reference | Study details |
|---|---|---|
| $FEV_1$ <2 l and age >60 years | Boushy et al (1971) | • Prospective study, 1964–1968<br>• $N = 142$ (all male)<br>• Various lung resections |
| ppo$FEV_1$ <0.8 l | Olsen et al (1975) | • Prospective study, $N = 56$<br>• $FEV_1$<0.8 l established on the basis of personal experience and observation of the level of activity of daily living (Gass and Olsen, 1986) |
| ppo$FEV_1$ <30% of normal | Gass and Olsen (1986) | • $N = 13$ (12 male), age 51–77 years<br>• Pneumonectomy in all cases |
| ppo$FEV_1$<40% of normal | Markos et al (1989) | • Prospective study, 1985–1986<br>• $N = 55$ (36 male), age 14–80 years<br>• Pneumonectomy, lobectomy or thoracotomy only; no surgery in two cases |
| DLCO <60% of predicted | Ferguson et al (1988) | • Prospective study, 1980–1987<br>• $N = 237$ (144 male), age 17–84 years (DLCO measurement: $N = 165$)<br>• Various lung resections |

complications. Hence, these tests cannot simply be compared with each other. Furthermore, the definitions of a 'medical complication' and of a 'pulmonary complication' remained unclear in this overview. Second, the calculation of multifactorial indices, such as the PPP or the PRQ, is interesting and appears to be simple. However, it is questionable both from the mathematical and the practicable point of view. Algebraic products of predicted lung function parameters (PPP: multiplication of the percentage ppo$FEV_1$ with the percentage post-operative predicted DLCO (ppoDLCO)) are used, and probability curves for complications are drawn (Pierce et al, 1994; Barrera and Melendez, 1996). However, the accuracy of these post-operative predicted values has been questioned. Bolliger et al (1996) showed that the time interval of the analysis (3 or 6 months after operation) is crucial: in this study a significant improvement was observed in all tests (spirometry, diffusion capacity and exercise testing) 6 months after lobectomy or pneumonectomy. In addition, in this investigation and in a study by Larsen et al (1997b) conventional pre-operative lung function testing overestimated the functional loss after lung resection. Hence, a possible inaccuracy inherently present in each of these tests may be amplified by multiplying two or more of these results. Above all, it is very delicate to implement the data obtained from such complications probability curves. What is the acceptable risk of post-operative complications and who should decide about cut-off values?

**Table 5.** Discriminative power to predict outcome: three predictive value groups (Zibrak et al, 1990; Melendez and Fischer, 1997).

| Group, predictive value | Test | Sensitivity | Specificity |
|---|---|---|---|
| A, poor predictor | Spirometry | 0.18 | 0.89 |
| | Spirometry blood gas analysis | 0.20 | 0.77 |
| | Stair climbing | 0.18 | 0.98 |
| B, intermediate predictor | Diffusion capacity | 0.67 | 0.72 |
| | Exercise-induced $SaO_2$ decrease | 0.43 | 0.90 |
| | Exercise PVR | 1.0 | 0.79 |
| C, good predictor | Predictive post-operative product (PPP) | 0.75 | 0.85 |
| | $VO_2$ max | 0.63 | 0.95 |
| | $VO_2$ max at 40 W | 0.83 | 0.95 |
| | Pulmonary respiratory quotient (PRQ) | 1.0 | 1.0 |

$SaO_2$, arterial oxygen saturation.

## Lung volume reduction surgery

In recent years, LVRS has been re-introduced in clinical practice to improve exercise tolerance and to relieve dyspnoea in patients with severe, end-stage pulmonary emphysema. On the basis of the work pioneered by Brantigan et al (1959) and on their own experience with lung transplantation in COPD patients, Cooper et al (1995) performed multiple wedge resections of the most severely affected emphysematous lung tissue in patients with diffuse pulmonary emphysema (mean $FEV_1$, 0.77 l=25% of predicted; residual lung volume, 5.9 l=288% of predicted). They used a median sternotomy as a surgical approach to both lungs, aiming at reducing total lung volume, and hence improving elastic recoil by improving radial traction on the airways. This concept proved to be successful: mean $FEV_1$ improved by 82%, and elevated pre-operative lung volumes decreased significantly (Cooper et al, 1995). In contrast to the considerable mortality (18%, i.e. six deaths out of 33 patients) reported by Brantigan et al (1959) some 35 years ago, there was no early or late mortality in the 20 patients of the series of Cooper et al (1995). Similar results were subsequently reported by others who used video-assisted thoracoscopy as a surgical approach to unilateral or bilateral LVRS (Bingisser et al, 1996; Keenan et al, 1996). The anaesthesiological methods included one-lung ventilation, use of thoracic epidural analgesia, tolerance of intra-operative hypercapnia and immediate post-operative tracheal extubation (Krucylak et al, 1996; Triantafillou, 1996; Zollinger et al, 1997; Zollinger and Pasch, 1998).

The concept of LVRS, i.e. (bilateral) lung resection in patients with pre-operative $FEV_1$ <0.8 l, the use of thoracoscopy with one-lung ventilation and immediate post-operative extubation in these patients following pulmonary resection, appears to contradict most previously established opinions and standards of thoracic surgery and anaesthesia. Indeed, hundreds of patients have successfully been treated and a huge number of papers have been published on this topic. However, many aspects of this new therapeutic modality remain to be elucidated. The different authors used similar, but not identical, principles of patient evaluation for LVRS (Bingisser et al, 1996; Yusen et al, 1996). Accordingly, there is no final consensus on the selection criteria for LVRS. In various reports, the conventional lung function parameters did not correlate significantly with objective outcome measures following LVRS (Bingisser et al, 1996; Brenner et al, 1997; Ingenito et al, 1998). McKenna et al (1997) reported that the presence of a bilateral upper lobe heterogenous pattern of emphysema on chest computed tomograpy and lung perfusion scans was the most important predictor of a favourable clinical outcome. Also, in patients studied by Weder et al (1997), the radiological emphysema morphology was associated with outcome after LVRS. Wisser et al (1998) recently presented a morphological grading system which would allow quantification and hence comparison of results between different patient groups and different therapeutic concepts. With regard to outcome prediction after LVRS, a number of alternative pulmonary function parameters other than classical lung function assessment have been described recently and appear to reflect better the changes associated with surgery. The ratio of residual volume (RV) to total lung capacity (TLC), RV/TLC, appears to be a major determinant of airflow limitation and was the single most important parameter of improvement in lung function following LVRS in a study by Fessler and Permutt (1998). Elastic recoil pressure significantly increased after LVRS (Sciurba et al, 1996). Ingenito et al (1998) stated that pre-operative measurement of inspiratory lung resistance may be useful to select patients suitable for LVRS. Furthermore, breathing characteristics, predominantly diaphragmatic function, appear to be essential for the effects of LVRS: Bloch et al (1997) suggested that a pre-operatively increased abdominal contribution to tidal volume may be associated with good results after LVRS and hence may be used for outcome prediction. Indeed, Benditt et al (1997) described significant changes in ventilatory muscle recruitment following LVRS, i.e. a greater contribution of the diaphragm and decreased use of intercostal and abdominal muscles during inspiration. Laghi et al (1998) found that the diaphragmatic neuromechanical coupling increased after surgery, that this was directly correlated with an increase in exercise capacity and that it was also related to a relief of dyspnoea.

Recent reports suggest that the limits for operability in patients with severe pulmonary emphysema have not yet been reached. Eugene et al (1997) performed LVRS successfully in 44 patients with a mean pre-operative $FEV_1$ of 0.41 l (range 0.23–0.50 l). Subjective improvement of dyspnoea was noted by 89% patients; mean $FEV_1$ and mean FVC increased by 51% and 56%, respectively. There was only one death within 30 days post-operatively in this study. Furthermore, LVRS was performed in long-term ventilator-dependent COPD patients, who were then successfully weaned from the ventilator and discharged home (Criner et al, 1996; Schmid et al, 1998). In lung transplant candidates with end-stage pulmonary emphysema, LVRS was used as an alternative to transplantation (Zenati et al, 1996). Finally, the concept of LVRS may also be applied in patients with severe pulmonary emphysema and lung cancer: 'Surgical treatment for lung cancer is now possible for patients who, prior to LVRS, had inoperable conditions due to poor pulmonary function' (McKenna et al, 1996).

In summary, the experience with LVRS indicates that conventional, so-called prohibitive lung function parameters should no longer be used to deny a potentially curative treatment or a surgical therapy which would significantly increase the quality of life. Low $FEV_1$ is more likely to be a symptom of present pulmonary impairment than an outcome predictor. Alternatively, more significant parameters of peri-operative morbidity and mortality need to be identified and verified. Serious outcome prediction will only be possible on the basis of large multicentre trials, which still have to be performed. An interdisciplinary approach to the specific problems of a severely compromised or co-morbid patient appears to be mandatory, because evidence-based data are not available for patients with impaired pulmonary function. The methods and concepts of modern anaesthesia, surgery and intensive care medicine are highly interrelated. Any further development in one specialty will influence the other. Therefore, continuous evolution in this field should be accompanied by a continuous re-evaluation of indications, contraindications, limitations and conventions.

## REFERENCES

American Thoracic Society (1987) Standardization of spirometry—1987 update. Statement of the American Thoracic Society. *American Review of Respiratory Disease* **136:** 1285–1298.

Barrera R & Melendez J (1996) Pulmonary respiratory quotient (PRQ) predicts pulmonary complications after thoracic surgery. *Chest* **110:** 215S (abstract).

Beaumont A, Cockroft A & Guz A (1985) A self-paced treadmill walking test for breathless patients. *Thorax* **40:** 459–465.

Bechard D & Wetstein L (1987) Assessment of exercise oxygen consumption as preoperative criterion for lung resection. *Annals of Thoracic Surgery* **44:** 344–349.

Benditt JO, Wood DE, McCool FD et al (1997) Changes in breathing and ventilatory muscle recruitment patterns induced by lung volume reduction surgery. *American Journal of Respiratory and Critical Care Medicine* **155:** 279–284.

Bernstein ML, Despars JA, Singh NP et al (1994) Reanalysis of the 12-minute walk in patients with chronic obstructive pulmonary disease. *Chest* **105:** 163–167.

*Bingisser R, Zollinger A, Hauser M et al (1996) Bilateral volume reduction surgery for diffuse pulmonary emphysema by video-assisted thoracoscopy. *Journal of Thoracic and Cardiovascular Surgery* **112:** 875–882.

Bloch KE, Li Y, Zhang J et al (1997) Effect of surgical lung volume reduction on breathing patterns in severe pulmonary emphysema. *American Journal of Respiratory and Critical Care Medicine* **156:** 553–560.

Bluman LG, Mosca L, Newman N et al (1998) Preoperative smoking habits and pulmonary complications. *Chest* **113:** 883–889.

Bolliger CT, Jordan P, Solèr M et al (1996) Pulmonary function and exercise capacity after lung resection. *European Respiratory Journal* **9:** 415–421.

Bolton JWR, Weiman DS, Haynes JL et al (1987) Stair climbing as an indicator of pulmonary function. *Chest* **92:** 783–788.

Boushy SF, Billig DM, North LB et al (1971) Clinical course related to preoperative and postoperative pulmonary function in patients with bronchogenic carcinoma. *Chest* **59:** 383–391.

Boysen PG, Block AJ, Olsen GN et al (1977) Prospective evaluation for pneumonectomy using $^{99m}$technetium quantitative perfusion lung scan. *Chest* **72:** 422–425.

Brantigan OC, Mueller E & Kress MB (1959) A surgical approach to pulmonary emphysema. *American Review of Respiratory Disease* **80:** 194–202.

Brenner M, McKenna R, Gelb A et al (1997) Objective predictors of response for staple versus laser emphysematous lung reduction. *American Journal of Respiratory and Critical Care Medicine* **155:** 1295–1301.

*Brooks-Brunn JA (1997) Predictors of postoperative pulmonary complications following abdominal surgery. *Chest* **111:** 564–571.

Cerfolio RJ, Allen MS, Trastek VF et al (1996) Lung resection in patients with compromised pulmonary function. *Annals of Thoracic Surgery* **62:** 348–351.

*Cooper JD, Trulock EP, Triantafillou AN et al (1995) Bilateral pneumectomy (volume reduction) for chronic obstructive pulmonary disease. *Journal of Thoracic and Cardiovascular Surgery* **109:** 106–119.

Cotes JE, Chinn DJ, Quanjer PH et al (1993) Report of the working party: standardization of lung function tests; European Community for Steel and Coal. Official Statement of the European Respiratory Society. Standardization of the measurement of transfer factor (diffusing capacity). *European Respiratory Journal* **6 (supplement):** 41–52.

Criner GJ, O'Brien G, Furukawa S et al (1996) Lung volume reduction surgery in ventilator-dependent COPD patients. *Chest* **110:** 877–884.

*Domino KB (1998) Anesthesia for the respiratory cripple. In Breen PH (ed.) *Respiration in Anesthesia: Pathophysiology and Clinical Update*, Anesthesiology Clinics of North America, vol. 16, pp 295–312. Philadelphia, PA: WB Saunders.

Eugene J, Dajee A, Kayaleh R et al (1997) Reduction pneumoplasty for patients with a forced expiratory volume in 1 second of 500 milliliters or less. *Annals of Thoracic Surgery* **63:** 186–192.

Ferguson MK, Little L, Rizzo L et al (1988) Diffusing capacity predicts morbidity and mortality after pulmonary resection. *Journal of Thoracic and Cardiovascular Surgery* **96:** 894–900.

Fessler HE & Permutt S (1998) Lung volume reduction surgery and airflow limitation. *American Journal of Respiratory and Critical Care Medicine* **157:** 715–722.

Gaensler EA, Cugell DW, Lindgren I et al (1954) The role of pulmonary insufficiency in mortality and invalidism following surgery for pulmonary tuberculosis. *Journal of Thoracic Surgery* **24:** 163–187.

Gass GD & Olsen GN (1986) Preoperative pulmonary function testing to predict postoperative morbidity and mortality. *Chest* **89:** 127–135.

Gift AG & Narsavage G (1998) Validity of the numeric rating scale as a measure of dyspnea. *American Journal of Critical Care* **7:** 200–204.

Hall JC, Tarala RA & Hall JL (1996) Respiratory insufficiency after abdominal surgery. *Respirology* **1:** 133–138.

*Ingenito EP, Evans RB, Loring SH et al (1998) Relation between preoperative inspiratory lung resistance and the outcome of lung-volume-reduction surgery for emphysema. *New England Journal of Medicine* **338:** 1181–1185.

Juhl B & Frost N (1975) A comparison between measured and calculated changes in the lung function after operation for pulmonary cancer. *Acta Anaesthesiologica Scandinavica* **57 (supplement):** 39–45.

Kearney DJ, Lee TH, Reilly JJ et al (1994) Assessment of operative risk in patients undergoing lung resection. Importance of predicted pulmonary function. *Chest* **105:** 753–759.

Keenan RJ, Landreneau RJ, Sciurba FC et al (1996) Unilateral thoracoscopic surgical approach for diffuse emphysema. *Journal of Thoracic and Cardiovascular Surgery* **111:** 308–316.

Krucylak PE, Naunheim KS, Keller CA et al (1996) Anesthetic management of patients undergoing unilateral video-assisted lung reduction for treatment of end-stage emphysema. *Journal of Cardiothoracic and Vascular Anesthesia* **10:** 850–853.

Laghi F, Jubran A, Topeli A et al (1998) Effect of lung volume reduction surgery on neuromechanical coupling of the diaphragm. *American Journal of Respiratory and Critical Care Medicine* **157:** 475–483.

Larsen KR, Lund JO, Svendsen UG et al (1997a) Prediction of post-operative cardiopulmonary function using perfusion scintigraphy in patients with bronchogenic carcinoma. *Clinical Physiology* **17:** 257–267.

Larsen KR, Svendsen UG, Milman N et al (1997b) Cardiopulmonary function at rest and during exercise after resection for bronchial carcinoma. *Annals of Thoracic Surgery* **64:** 960–964.

*Lawrence VA, Dhanda R, Hilsenbeck SG & Page CP (1996) Risk of pulmonary complications after elective abdominal surgery. *Chest* **110:** 744–750.

McCulloch TM, Jensen NF, Girod DA et al (1997) Risk factors for pulmonary complications in the postoperative head and neck surgery patient. *Head and Neck* **19:** 372–377.

McGavin CR, Gupta SP & McHardy GJR (1976) Twelve-minute walking test for assessing disability in chronic bronchitis. *British Medical Journal* **1:** 822–823.

McKenna RJ, Fischel RJ, Brenner M et al (1996) Combined operations for lung volume reduction surgery and lung cancer. *Chest* **110:** 885–888.

McKenna RJ, Brenner M, Fischel RJ et al (1997) Patient selection criteria for lung volume reduction surgery. *Journal of Thoracic and Cardiovascular Surgery* **114:** 957–964.

Mahler DA, Weinberg DH, Wells CK & Feinstein AR (1984) The measurement of dyspnea: contents, interobserver agreement, and physiologic correlates of two new clinical indexes. *Chest* **85:** 751–758.

Markos J, Mullan BP, Hillman DR et al (1989) Preoperative assessment as a predictor of mortality and morbidity after lung resection. *American Review of Respiratory Disease* **139:** 902–910.

*Melendez JA & Fischer ME (1997) Preoperative pulmonary evaluation of the thoracic surgical patient. In Wilson RS (ed.) *Anesthesia*, Chest Surgery Clinics of North America, vol. 7, pp 641–654. Philadelphia, PA: WB Saunders.

Miller JI, Grossman GD & Hatcher CR (1981) Pulmonary function test criteria for operability and pulmonary resection. *Surgery, Gynecology and Obstetrics* **153:** 893–895.

*Mitchell CK, Smoger SH, Pfeifer MP et al (1998) Multivariate analysis of factors associated with postoperative pulmonary complications following general elective surgery. *Archives of Surgery* **133:** 194–198.

Mittman C (1961) Assessment of operative risk in thoracic surgery. *American Review of Respiratory Disease* **84:** 197–207.

Neuhaus H & Cherniak N (1968) A bronchospirometric method of estimating the effect of pneumonectomy on the maximal breathing capacity. *Journal of Thoracic and Cardiovascular Surgery* **55:** 144–148.

Van Nostrand D, Kjelsberg MO & Humphrey EW (1968) Preresectional evaluation of risk for pneumonectomy. *Surgery, Gynecology and Obstetrics* **127:** 306–312.

Olsen GN, Block AJ, Swenson EW et al (1975) Pulmonary function evaluation of the lung resection candidate: a prospective study. *American Review of Respiratory Disease* **111:** 379–387.

Pierce RJ, Copland JM, Sharpe K et al (1994) Preoperative risk evaluation for lung cancer resection: predicted postoperative product as a predictor of surgical mortality. *American Journal of Respiratory and Critical Care Medicine* **150:** 947–955.

Quanjer PH, Tammeling GJ, Pederson OF et al (1993) Report of the working party: standardization of lung function tests; European Community for Steel and Coal. Official Statement of the

European Respiratory Society. Lung volumes and forced ventilatory flows. *European Respiratory Journal* **6 (supplement):** 5–40.

Rady MY, Ryan T & Starr NJ (1997) Early onset of acute pulmonary dysfunction after cardiovascular surgery: risk factors and clinical outcome. *Critical Care Medicine* **25:** 1831–1839.

Reilly JJ, Mentzer SJ & Sugarbaker DJ (1993) Preoperative assessment of patients undergoing pulmonary resection. *Chest* **103 (supplement):** 342–345.

Schmid RA, Vogt P, Stocker R et al (1998) Lung volume reduction surgery for a patient receiving mechanical ventilation after a complex cardiac operation. *Journal of Thoracic and Cardiovascular Surgery* **115:** 236–237.

Sciurba FC, Rogers RM, Keenan RJ et al (1996) Improvement in pulmonary function and elastic recoil after lung-reduction surgery for diffuse emphysema. *New England Journal of Medicine* **334:** 1095–1099.

Task Group on Screening for Respiratory Disease in Occupational Settings (1982) Official Statement of the American Thoracic Society. *American Review of Respiratory Disease* **126:** 952–956.

Triantafillou AN (1996) Anesthetic management for bilateral volume reduction surgery. *Seminars in Thoracic and Cardiovascular Surgery* **8:** 94–98.

Weder W, Thurnheer R, Stammberger U et al (1997) Radiologic emphysema morphology is associated with outcome after surgical lung volume reduction. *Annals of Thoracic Surgery* **64:** 313–319.

Weiner P, Zeidan F, Zamir D et al (1998) Prophylactic inspiratory muscle training in patients undergoing coronary artery bypass graft. *World Journal of Surgery* **22:** 427–431.

Wisser W, Klepetko W, Kontrus M et al (1998) Morphologic grading of the emphysematous lung and its relation to improvement after lung volume reduction surgery. *Annals of Thoracic Surgery* **65:** 793–799.

*Wong DH, Weber EC, Schell MJ et al (1995) Factors associated with postoperative pulmonary complications in patients with severe chronic obstructive pulmonary disease. *Anesthesia and Analgesia* **80:** 276–284.

Yusen RD, Lefrak SS & Washington University Emphysema Surgery Group (1996) Evaluation of patients with emphysema for lung volume reduction surgery. *Seminars in Thoracic and Cardiovascular Surgery* **8:** 83–93.

Zenati M, Keenan RJ, Sciurba FC et al (1996) Role of lung reduction in lung transplant candidates with pulmonary emphysema. *Annals of Thoracic Surgery* **62:** 994–999.

Zibrak JD, O'Donnell CR & Marton K (1990) Indications for pulmonary testing. *Annals of Internal Medicine* **112:** 673–771.

Zollinger A & Pasch T (1998) Anaesthesia for lung volume reduction surgery. *Current Opinion in Anaesthesiology* **11:** 45–49.

*Zollinger A, Zaugg M, Weder W et al (1997) Video-assisted thoracoscopic volume reduction surgery in patients with diffuse pulmonary emphysema: gas exchange and anesthesiological management. *Anesthesia and Analgesia* **84:** 845–851.

6

# The patient under chronic medication

PIERRE CORIAT MD, FANZCA

Professor and Chairman

LOUISE GOUILLE MD

Staff Anaesthesiologist

*Groupe Hospitalier Pitié-Salpêtrière, 47–83 Boulevard de l'Hôpital, 75651 Paris Cedex 13, France*

Most high-risk patients scheduled for surgery benefit from treatment designed to improve both their symptoms and their life expectancy. Cardiovascular treatments interfere with regulatory mechanisms of blood pressure and regional circulations, or they affect the cardiac electrophysiology and contractility. This explains why most peri-operative circulatory abnormalities are not due to the effect of anaesthetic agents on the circulation but to the interactions between cardiovascular and anaesthetic agents, both of which alter the functioning of several physiological systems. On the other hand, when given peri-operatively, some treatments are effective in blunting the circulatory response to surgical stimulation and post-operative stress. In this chapter we describe the interactions between treatments chronically taken by high-risk patients and anaesthesia. This subject makes one look at-physiology and pharmacology and allows a better understanding of the compensatory mechanisms activated in response to the stress of surgery and anaesthesia.

**Key words:** cardiovascular agents; pharmacology; peri-operative management; renin–angiotensin system; hypertension; hypotension.

## β-ADRENOCEPTOR ANTAGONISTS

It is now widely accepted that patients chronically treated with β-blockers should undergo surgery with a well-controlled blood pressure, and that this therapy must be maintained up to the day of surgery and restored as soon as possible thereafter (Waltier, 1998). This consensus arises from the evidence that the continuation of β-adrenoceptors in the pre-operative period provides well-established beneficial effects, including the prevention of hypertension, dysrhythmias and myocardial ischaemia (Roizen, 1988; Stone et al, 1988).

*Baillière's Clinical Anaesthesiology*—
Vol. 12, No. 3, September 1998
ISBN 0–7020–2536–4
0950–3501/98/030405 + 14 $12.00/00

The use of β-blockers with anaesthesia limits the haemodynamic response to nociceptive stimuli which characterize the peri-operative period: tracheal intubation, surgical stimulation and metabolic stress due to the recovery period. In addition it is firmly established that β-blockers, given with pre-medication, do not increase the lowering blood pressure effect of anaesthesia (Still et al, 1985; Stone et al, 1988). The effects of β-blockers on contractility are cumulative with those of anaesthetic agents and there is no potentiation. In vascular surgical patients, suffering from poorly controlled hypertension, the pre-operative administration of β-blockers was effective in blunting the increase in blood pressure and heart rate, and in preventing myocardial ischaemia associated with intubation and the recovery period (Stone et al, 1988).

The beneficial effects of β-blockers on myocardial oxygen balance explain why, in patients suffering from coronary artery disease, when they are administered intravenously and then orally as soon as abdominal transit has resumed they improve outcome following surgery. In a recent study, prophylactic β-blocking therapy was given throughout the operative period to patients with coronary risk factors (Mangano et al, 1996). Continuous electrocardiogram recordings with the Holter method confirmed that the administration of atenolol decreased by half the incidence of post-operative myocardial ischaemia (Wallace et al, 1998). Whereas the incidence of post-operative complications observed on leaving the hospital did not differ in patients receiving β-blockers versus the placebo group of patients, the occurrence of coronary complications in the year following surgery was significantly decreased in the group of patients receiving β-blockers peri-operatively and during the week of surgery. The follow-up of patients 2 years after the operation showed a higher survival rate in those having received atenolol: 90% compared with 79% in the placebo group. Furthermore a larger percentage of patients were free from cardiovascular incident in the treated group (83% versus 68%) (Mangano et al, 1996). Therefore, interactions between β-blockers and circulatory response to anaesthesia and surgery are much more beneficial than deleterious. The surgical patients fully benefit from the positive effects of this medication on myocardial oxygen balance without any threat to their circulatory system. The beneficial effects appear to improve the cardiac risk of anaesthesia in the medium and long term. For all these reasons it is imperative that a surgical patient being treated with a β-blocker receive this together with his or her pre-medication. The risk of myocardial ischaemia that may accompany the discontinuation of β-blocker treatment is an additional reason to continue the treatment until the morning of surgery.

However, it should be remembered that the administration of β-blockers during pre-medication or during anaesthesia limits the adaptation of cardiac output to the metabolic needs which are markedly increased during the recovery. Prophylactic administration of β-blockers must not be considered until left ventricle function of the patient has been checked by a clinical examination and, if necessary, by means of complementary examinations, such as echocardiography or isotopic angioscintigraphy, which give an objective and reliable evaluation of left ventricular function.

## ANGIOTENSIN-CONVERTING ENZYME INHIBITORS

Angiotensin-converting enzyme (ACE) inhibitors (ACEIs) are increasingly used in the treatment of cardiovascular or other diseases (Gavras, 1990). The number of patients chronically treated with ACEIs and scheduled for anaesthesia is increasing and the question arises of whether renin–angiotensin system (RAS) blockade may affect haemodynamics during anaesthesia and surgery. Although anaesthesia is not invariably associated with deleterious haemodynamic events in ACE-blocked patients, haemodynamic instability manifest as unexpected episodes of hypotension has been described in these patients (Mirenda and Grissom, 1991). Recent advances in RAS physiology and ACEI pharmacology may help in understanding the haemodynamic risks of anaesthesia in the ACE-blocked patient, in identifying some predisposing factors, and in determining the potential beneficial effects of ACE inhibition during anaesthesia and surgery.

The sympathetic nervous system and the RAS are the two principal components which regulate the arterial blood pressure. These systems play an important role during the operative period in the regulation of the haemodynamic constraints brought on by anaesthesia, surgical stimuli and peri-operative blood loss (Miller et al, 1978a,b). While the sympathetic system is for the most part activated by nociceptive stimulations such as intubation and surgery the RAS is activated by any decrease in venous return which lowers pre-load, such as hypovolaemia, or the effect of anaesthetic drugs or spinal anaesthesia. That explains why the arterial blood pressure of patients chronically treated with ACEIs is characterized by volume dependence (Gavras, 1990). In the course of animal experimentations and studies done on healthy volunteers, blockade of the RAS significantly increases the lowering blood pressure effect of both spinal and general anaesthesia (Figure 1). The blood pressure decrease was greater if anaesthesia was maintained with volatile anaesthetic agents and significantly more pronounced in the case of hypovolaemia (Miller et al, 1978a,b).

ACEI therapy has specific effects on the loading conditions of the heart and the autonomic system. Vasodilatation involves both resistance and capacitance vessels (Vidt et al, 1982; Todd and Heel, 1986). It is important to take into account the veinodilatation due to ACEIs when considering the mechanisms by which these agents interfere with the immediate regulation of systemic haemodynamics at induction of anaesthesia. The decreased tone in capacitance vessels accentuates the decrease in blood pressure provoked by induction through an increase in blood pooling at the expense of cardiac filling. This mechanism is enhanced by the presence of either a pre-operative hypovolaemia or altered left ventricular diastolic function, both frequently seen in old, hypertensive or vascular surgical patients.

In addition, chronic ACEI therapy increases vagal tone and interferes with the function of the sympathetic nervous system. In particular it attenuates adrenergic responsiveness in awake and anaesthetized patients (Kataja et al, 1989).

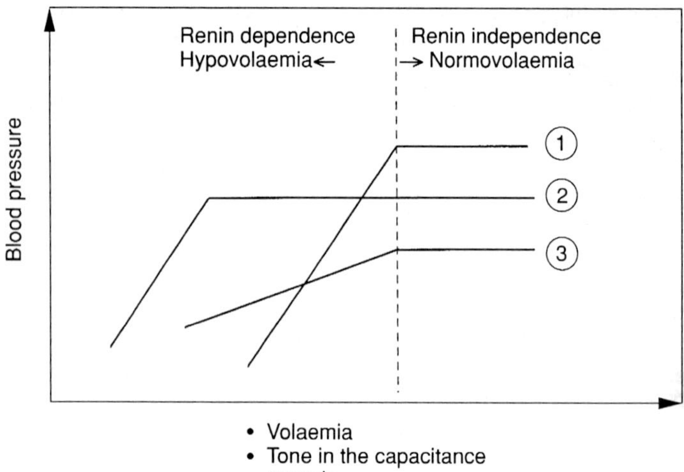


**Figure 1.** Relationship between plasma renin activity and effective volaemia: curve 1, hypertensive patient with ACEIs; curve 2, untreated patient; curve 3, patient with poor left ventricular function and ACEIs. In normovolaemic patients blood pressure is maintained without RAS activity. If the patient becomes hypovolaemic blood pressure is maintained by the two actions of angiotensin II: vasoconstriction of both resistance and capacitance vessels and volaemia restoration. In hypertensive patients treated with ACEIs, blood pressure becomes volaemia dependent, because no compensatory mechanism counteracts hypovolaemia. In these patients any decrease in venous return markedly interferes with stroke volume, and consequently a marked decrease in blood pressure often results from hypovolaemia.

## Pre-operative treatment with angiotensin-converting enzyme inhibitors: continue or discontinue?

To determine whether ACE inhibition therapy should be continued up to the day of the surgical procedure, a standard practice for other modern antihypertensive agents, it should be known whether stopping the treatment does or does not lead to a hypertensive episode before surgery or at intubation and whether continuing treatment is or is not associated with an unacceptable fall in blood pressure at induction.

Data from the literature (Kataja et al, 1989; Colson et al, 1992; Coriat et al, 1994) obtained in patients chronically treated with ACEIs treated for hypertension or left ventricular dysfunction demonstrate that (1) withdrawal of ACEI therapy before surgery does not result in a higher incidence of either hypertensive episodes or congestive heart failure both preoperatively and at intubation, (2) the temporary withdrawal of ACEIs does not lead to an abnormal blood pressure response to induction and intubation and (3) in hypertensive patients who received ACEIs together with their pre-medication, the lowering blood pressure effect of anaesthesia is increased, leading to an increased need for vasopressive agents to maintain blood pressure.

There is no 'rebound syndrome' when ACEI treatment is discontinued. At most, the myocardial function and blood pressure will return to the previous level (Vidt et al, 1982; Todd and Heel, 1986). It appears that, in the case of discontinued treatment 24 or 48 hours before surgery, there will be no risk of a hypertensive episode (Coriat et al, 1994; Pflugfelder et al, 1995) or congestive heart failure (Pflugfelder et al, 1995). Two facts may account for the lack of deleterious events associated with the pre-operative withdrawal of ACEIs. First, after temporary interruption of a chronic ACEI treatment, tissue ACE inhibition although less pronounced persists for several days. Second, chronic ACEI treatment exerts long-lasting beneficial effects on the structural and/or functional vascular and myocardial alterations (Gavras, 1990).

The administration of ACEIs before surgery does not limit a hypertensive episode caused by nociceptive stimuli (intubation or surgery) and moreover they do not prevent them (Kataja et al, 1989; Colson et al, 1992; Coriat et al, 1994). As part of a routine clinical practice, the patient's usual anti-hypertensive treatment is given before surgery. When ACEIs were introduced, this approach was followed in patients receiving these drugs. Exaggerated hypotensive responses to induction and maintenance of anaesthesia leading in many cases to severe hypotension have been reported (Kataja et al, 1989; Colson et al, 1992; Coriat et al, 1994). Low cerebral blood flow associated with low mean arterial pressure has been demonstrated in anaesthetized patients treated with captopril but not in those receiving a β-adrenoceptor blocker (Jensen et al, 1989).

Two controlled studies confirmed that in hypertensive patients chronically treated with ACEIs, therapy up to the day of surgery is a major factor influencing blood pressure responsiveness to induction (Colson et al, 1992; Coriat et al, 1994). If enalapril therapy was continued, a very low plasma converting enzyme activity was be observed and an exaggerated hypotensive response occurred at induction (Coriat et al, 1994). If captopril therapy is continued, the magnitude of the decrease in blood pressure in response to induction, although lower than with enalapril, is enhanced compared with that noted in patients in whom captopril has been withheld (Table 1). The other factors that could significantly modify blood pressure are a high dose of captopril (>100 mg/day) or enalapril (>10 mg/day), diastolic left ventricle dysfunction, renal failure, hypovolaemia or hypothermia during the operative period.

**Table 1.** Plasma converting enzyme activity (normal value: 27 nmol/ml per min) and arterial blood pressure measured after induction in patients treated with captopril or enalapril for essential hypertension.

| | Treatment continued | | Treatment discontinued | |
|---|---|---|---|---|
| | Enalapril | Captopril | Enalapril | Captopril |
| ACE activity (nmol/ml per min) | 2.5 ± 2.3 | 11.1 ± 5.0 | 12.4 ± 8.3 | 22.5 ± 5.0 |
| Systolic arterial pressure (mmHg) | 71 ± 10 | 86 ± 11 | 100 ± 15 | 101 ± 21 |
| Percentage of patients who needed vasopressor after induction | 100 | 18 | 63 | 20 |

Blood pressure is lower when patients received enalapril than captopril the morning before surgery. Blood pressure decrease is significantly less if treatment has not been administered the morning of surgery (according to Coriat et al, 1994).

For all these reasons, it is preferable not to continue ACEI therapy up to the day of surgery in hypertensive patients. If therapy is continued special attention must be paid to maintaining an adequate volume loading throughout the peri-operative period and to using vasopressor therapy when needed to maintain blood pressure.

Because of arterial–ventricular coupling, the anaesthesia blood pressure regulation would be different when patients received ACEIs for arterial hypertension or for congestive heart failure (Ryckwaert and Colson, 1997). In patients suffering from hypertension usually associated with relatively low blood volume and impaired left ventricle diastolic function, any decrease, even moderate, in venous return in response to anaesthesia or to a hypovolaemic stress leads to a major decrease in arterial blood pressure. By contrast, in a patient with chronic heart failure due to altered contractility the decrease in venous tone is much better tolerated and the decrease in afterload from ACEI treatment improves left ventricular function and output.

In chronic heart failure, the beneficial effects of ACE inhibition include increased cardiac output and left ventricular function, improved myocardial oxygen balance and reduced incidence of atrial and ventricular arrhythmia (SOLVD Investigators, 1991). However, potential adverse effects of ACE inhibition must be taken into account: peri-operative hypotension, which may be difficult to counteract because of the lower vasopressor effect of sympathetic agonist agents (Licker et al, 1996). The dose of norepinephrine that must be administered in order to obtain a 20% increase in blood pressure during anaesthesia is twice as high if the patient has long-term ACEI treatment. When hypotension is unresponsive to this therapy, an agonist of the arginin vasopressin system is highly effective in restoring blood pressure.

In conclusion, recommendations to continue hypertensive treatment until the day of surgery are justified when calcium blocking agents or β-blockers are administered but cannot be extrapolated in the case of patients treated with ACEIs. In hypertensive patients chronically treated with ACEIs, therapy up to the day of surgery is a major factor influencing blood pressure responsiveness to general or epidural anaesthesia. By contrast, in patients suffering from left ventricular dysfunction chronically treated with ACEIs, it may be worth continuing the chronic treatment with ACEIs which might improve left ventricular function. However, the treatment can be stopped without worsening the circulatory status. In these patients, to withdraw ACEIs pre-operatively would allow recovery of RAS control of blood pressure but at the expense of left ventricular function. The evidence is that even in these patients ACE inhibition does not allow the anaesthesiologist to be tolerant of hypovolaemia.

### Angiotensin II receptor antagonists

A new class of anti-hypertensive drugs has recently emerged: the angiotensin II receptor antagonists such as losartan, valsartan and candesartan. The potential therapeutic interest of this group of drugs is twofold. First, they should not induce the bradykinin-related side-effects of ACEIs such as cough, which occurs in 10–20% of patients receiving ACEIs (Licker et al, 1996). Because bradykinin breakdown reduction by ACEIs could also participate in their haemodynamic effect, angiotensin II receptor antagonists may not provide a similar therapeutic profile. Second, because they competitively block angiotensin II receptors ($AT_1$), they should suppress angiotensin II effects better than ACEIs.

Clinical experience clearly shows that when this treatment is continued up to the day of surgery severe hypotensive episodes occur at induction and intra-operatively. This emphasizes the role and function of the RAS in maintaining intra-operative blood pressure stability and leads to the recommendation to stop the treatment at least 24 hours before surgery.

## CALCIUM CHANNEL BLOCKERS

The calcium blocking agents inhibit the transmembrane influx of calcium ions into cardiac and vascular smooth muscle (Braunwald, 1982). They relax vascular smooth muscle, decrease pacemaker activity and reduce cardiac muscle contractile force. However, they exhibit variable selectivity for inhibiting slow-channel calcium fluxes in vascular smooth muscle (Henry, 1980). Calcium blocking drugs cause primarily arterial vasodilatation. This effect reduces left ventricle afterload and may improve ventricular ejection. Pre-load usually changes little because venodilatation is minimal, and negative inotropy is often offset by reduced afterload. This explains why these medications show excellent tolerance when administered during the operative period.

Calcium channel blockers of the dihydropyridine group, nifedipine, nicardipine and nitrendipine, are widely prescribed for hypertension. These agents give vasodilatation which activates the baroreceptor reflex, causing sympathetic stimulation (Kiowski et al, 1986). This effect may be responsible for the potential deleterious effect of short-acting dihydropyridine, reported during long-term treatment in patients with coronary artery disease (Furberg et al, 1995).

The arterial vasodilatation effects of nifedipine with halothane are additive. The same is true for the combination of nicardipine with isoflurane. However, when halogenated agents are administered at high concentrations, the hypotensive effects of calcium inhibitors are proportionally more marked.

Verapamil is the calcium channel blocker which has the most pronounced negative inotropic effect (Kapur et al, 1984a,b). A potentiation risk exists with verapamil on myocardial depression when enflurane is used over 1 MAC (Kiowski et al, 1986). The negative inotropic effects of verapamil and halothane are additive. However, the addition of the negative inotropic effects of these two agents may result in a significant myocardial depression. This is the reason why isoflurane is recommended in patients treated with verapamil. With verapamil, the negative chronotropic effects of fentanyl and isoflurane are only additive (Kapur et al, 1984b). However, there exists a potentiation if enflurane is used over 1 MAC or if verapamil has been administered orally or intravenously so as to obtain a high plasmatic level (over 400 ng/ml). Oral pre-operative administration of diltiazem does not expose the patient to such bradycardia.

In the case of tachyarrhythmia verapamil and diltiazem administered intravenously during the peri-operative period, by their effect on nodal conduction, have high efficacy for slowing down heart rate. However, they do not restore sinus rhythm (Rinkenberger et al, 1980). Calcium channel blockers slightly increase the effect of muscle relaxants (Arndts, 1983). The clinical significance of these interactions is difficult to quantitate. With patients treated with verapamil, the dose of long-duration muscle relaxants administered should be reduced.

## $\alpha_2$-ADRENOCEPTOR AGONISTS

The $\alpha_2$-adrenoreceptor agonists have been used as anti-hypertensive medication for a long time. In fact, they have many other properties which are the result of the widespread distribution of the $\alpha_2$-adrenergic receptors in the body and their contributions to different physiological regulations (Arndts, 1983). Apart from their haemodynamic properties, which limit the acceleration of heart rate, and the increase in the loading condition of the heart which characterizes the post-operative period, another major property of the $\alpha_2$-adrenoceptor agonists is that of inducing sedation and providing analgesia, thus decreasing the overall metabolic post-operative stress (Muzi et al, 1992).

In the peri-operative period the $\alpha_2$-adrenoceptor agonists have a particularly marked beneficial effect, as they directly oppose step by step all the physiological mechanisms which may lead to the occurrence of heart failure or acute coronary complications (Muzi et al, 1992). In fact, they very successfully limit the increase in plasma catecholamines, control the rise in global oxygen consumption and spectacularly anticipate post-operative shivering (Flacke et al, 1987; Quintin et al, 1990, 1991, 1996) (Table 2). As a result, the incidence of episodes of post-operative ischaemia is significantly diminished with the administration of preventive $\alpha_2$-adrenoceptor agonists (Europe Research Group, 1997).

$\alpha_2$-Adrenoceptor agonists can be safety administered several days after surgery as they 'modulate' but do not totally block the sympathetic system and interfere little with the chronotropic, inotropic and vasopressor effects of its agonists (Muzi et al, 1992). Today, one of the limitations of their prophylactic administration is related to the duration of effect of clonidine, which is characterized by a long elimination half-life. This is why the two $\alpha_2$-adrenoreceptor agonists which are being developed (mivazerol (Europe Research Group, 1997) and dexmedetomidine (Atlee and Bosnjak, 1990)), and which have a much shorter half-life, appear in practice to be much better adapted to peri-operative administration (in continuous perfusion) in high-risk cardiac patients undergoing surgery.

**Table 2.** Haemodynamic modifications observed after vascular surgery in hypertensive patients treated with either clonidine or a placebo during the peri-operative period.

| | Placebo | Clonidine |
|---|---|---|
| Pre-operative period | | |
| Alfentanil total dose (μg/kg) | 144 ± 66 | 84 ± 51 |
| Isoflurane inspiratory fraction (%) | 0.72 ± 0.37 | 0.44 ± 0.28 |
| Post-operative period | | |
| Duration of post-operative mechanical ventilation/min | 111 ± 50 | 59 ± 61 |
| Number of tachycardia episodes | 1.6 ± 1.9 | 0.3 ± 0.6 |
| Duration of tachycardia episode (min) | 94 ± 82 | 5 ± 13 |
| Number of hypertensive episodes | 3 ± 2 | 1 ± 3 |
| Duration of hypertensive episode (min) | 64 ± 54 | 13 ± 27 |

Adapted from Quintin et al (1996, *Anesthesia and Analgesia* **83:** 687–695).

If the multicentre studies which are taking place at present demonstrate that mivazerol significantly limits post-operative cardiac complications and improves survival rate in patients with patent or suspected coronary artery disease, then we can envisage more extended administration of this new $\alpha_2$-adrenoreceptor agonist in order to decrease the incidence of post-operative cardiac complication in these individuals.

## ANTI-ARRHYTHMIC AGENTS

Particular attention must be paid when using halogenated volatile anaesthetic as the sole anaesthetic agent in patients under long-term treatment with class 1 anti-arrhythmic agents (Quintin et al, 1996). As both agents decrease atrioventricular conduction by two different mechanisms, there exists a risk of potentiation leading to heart block. Class 1A and 1C anti-arrhythmics which are membrane stabilizers significantly prolong the effect of muscle relaxants. This absolutely requires adaptation of muscle relaxant administration in these patients.

When a cardiologist prescribes an anti-arrhythmic agent, it is in order to avoid an episode of sudden death, an event that can be avoided if the patient is correctly monitored. Because anti-arrhythmics are administered to prevent arrhythmia, maintenance of anti-arrhythmic therapy during the peri-operative period appears suitable. The choice of the anaesthetic technique will be made by taking into consideration the effect of the anaesthetic agents on ventricular excitability and above all intracardiac conduction (Gallagher et al, 1986). However, an anti-arrhythmic agent is never 100% effective and, during the peri-operative period, sudden changes in heart rate, in the loading conditions of the heart or in cathecholergic secretion may increase the risk for auricular or ventricular arrhythmias (Woosley, 1991). A worsening of arrhythmias has been noted in 12% of a group of patients suffering from coronary artery disease undergoing major non-cardiac surgery (O'Kelly et al, 1992). However, this study does not conclude that an aggressive anti-arrhythmic treatment during the peri-operative period is necessary. When an anti-arrhythmic treatment has been prescribed for a non-sustained benign arrhythmia it seems preferable to withdraw the treatment during the operative period.

## ANTI-COAGULANT AND ANTI-PLATELET DRUGS

These medications are frequently prescribed for patients with vascular or coronary artery disease. When a patient under chronic treatment with these medications is scheduled for surgery a risk of increased bleeding coexists with the risk of not having an effective prevention for arterial coronary or venous thrombotic complications (Ferraris and Swanson, 1983; Bartley and Warndahl, 1992; Fauno et al, 1993). Importantly, in the presence of any drug which interferes with the coagulation system the use of epidural or intrathecal anaesthesia is contraindicated.

### Anti-coagulants

In patients suffering from chronic heart failure and under long-term oral anti-coagulant (OAC) therapy, the medication can be stopped several days before surgery. The use of OACs in the chronic heart failure patient is limited to those having atrial arrhythmia or to those whose echocardiogram has shown microthrombi in a dilated atrium. A recent study on thrombo-embolic accidents in chronic heart failure patients reveals that the risk of cerebral or peripheral embolism is low and not significantly reduced by anti-vitamin K (Davies et al, 1974).

In patients in whom it is essential to continue the anti-coagulant therapy, if surgery is scheduled a couple of days after their arrival in the surgical unit, switching to heparin (beware of the additional risk of haemorrhage) should be taken into consideration. After surgery, the oral anticoagulant treatment can be resumed easily if vitamin K has been used scarcely. If a patient treated with OACs must undergo surgery rapidly, the use of several drops (1–5 mg) of vitamin K given orally is generally sufficient to reach an index normalized ratio (INR) around 1.5 within 8 hours which would be enough to control an eventual risk of haemorrhage.

### Anti-platelet agents

These agents act on primary haemostasis (platelet–vascular wall interactions) and therefore interfere directly with surgical haemostasis (Davies et al, 1974; Ferraris and Swanson, 1983; Connely and Panush, 1991). They act by means of an irreversible cyclo-oxygenase acetylation and therefore by inhibition of thromboxane synthesis (aspirin or non-steroidal/anti-inflammatory drugs (NSAIDs)) or by inhibiting the adenosine diphosphate (ADP) route of activation (ticlopidine). Several basic elements which differentiate aspirin and NSAIDs from ticlopidine must be taken into account (Davies et al, 1974; Connely and Panush, 1991).

Aspirin-induced platelet inhibition may be observed with the lowest doses (30–40 mg). There is no argument suggesting that the risk of bleeding (other than haemorrhages from gastric lesions) is higher when the aspirin dose exceeds the minimal dose necessary to inhibit 95% of the thromboxane synthesis. Special attention must be paid to patients who receive aspirin as part of a treatment for coronary artery disease. In these patients, to withdraw aspirin may lead to coronary complications such as unstable angina or myocardial infarction. In these cases, aspirin must be continued until the day of surgery. If the surgical procedure does not allow for that, aspirin must be stopped a week before surgery and either NSAIDs or low-molecular-weight heparin must be given.

NSAIDs have the same target as aspirin but cyclo-oxygenase inhibition is reversible (the cyclo-oxygenase inhibition by aspirin is irreversible). Consequently, the anti-platelet effects of NSAIDs disappear a couple of hours after the withdrawal of the treatment (Conrad et al, 1988). This is why these agents appear to be an interesting substitute for aspirin during the pre-operative period when an anti-platelet agent is essential for the patient (Bartley and Warndahl, 1992).

The anti-haemostatic effects are clinically more pronounced with ticlopidine than with aspirin. This platelet aggregation inhibitor increases the bleeding time (at least twice its initial level) (Davies et al, 1974). There exists, however, a certain percentage of patients who, under the standard recommended dosage (250 mg twice per day), maintain a normal bleeding time.

## DIGITALIS

The problems posed by digitalis during the surgical period come, on the one hand, from the small margin between therapeutic and toxic concentrations of these agents (Williams et al, 1995) and, on the other, from the frequent electrolyte abnormalities during the peri-operative period. The lack of deleterious effect of temporary withdrawal of chronic digitalis therapy has been shown by studies performed in patients with chronic cardiac failure. A multicentre study conducted by Parker et al (1993) showed that interruption of the digitalis treatment is accompanied by a significant increase in the number of heart attacks and hospitalizations. However, the clinical state of the patient starts worsening only several weeks after the interruption of the treatment. More recently a multicentre study performed in patients suffering from congestive heart failure who received either digoxin or a placebo (Digitalis Investigation Group, 1997) showed that the death rate after 37 months from cardiac or extracardiac origin was not improved in those treated with digoxin. The fact that one can interrupt digitalis treatment for several days without worsening the circulatory condition of the patient and the potential toxicity of digitalis during the post-operative period lead to the conclusion that it is preferable to interrupt digitalis treatment for 2 or 3 days before surgery for patients with a congestive heart failure in sinus rhythm. In patients with atrial fibrillation, the digitalis treatment must be continued and pre-operative clinical assessment must ensure the absence of any signs indicating a digitalis intoxication.

## CONCLUSION

Some interactions between cardiovascular treatment and anaesthesia are undoubtedly beneficial because they improve peri-operative haemodynamic stability and myocardial oxygen balance. This is the case of β-blockers and calcium blocking agents whose treatment must be continued until the day of the surgery. Other interactions between agents which markedly limit the body compensatory mechanisms that come into force to maintain the circulatory balance during the peri-operative period may not be beneficial. This is true for ACEIs which, on the one hand, improve cardiac function but, on the other, have a potential adverse effect on blood pressure. For all agents, a thorough knowledge of the pharmacology of the medication administered and its repercussions on peri-operative haemodynamics allows for a logical attitude when considering the continuation or interruption of cardiovascular treatment.

## REFERENCES


Arndts D (1983) New aspects of the clinical pharmacology of clonidine. *Chest* **83:** 397–400.

Atlee JL III & Bosnjak ZJ (1990) Mechanisms for cardiac dysrhythmias during anesthesia. *Anesthesiology* **72:** 3437–3474.

Bartley GB & Warndahl RA (1992) Surgical bleeding associated with aspirin and nonsteroidal anti-inflammatory agents. *Mayo Clinic Proceedings* **67:** 402–403 (letter).

Braunwald E (1982) Mechanism of action of calcium-channel-blocking agents. *New England Journal of Medicine* **307:** 1618–1627.

Colson P, Saussine M, Seguin JR et al (1992) Hemodynamic effects of anesthesia in patients chronically treated with angiotensin-converting enzyme inhibitors. *Anesthesia and Analgesia* **74:** 805–808.

Connely CS & Panush RS (1991) Should non steroidal anti inflammatory drugs be stopped before elective surgery? *Archives of Internal Medicine* **151:** 1963–1966.

Conrad KA, Fagan TC, Mackie MJ & Mayshar PV (1988) Effects of ketorolac thrometamine on hemostasis in volunteers. *Clinical Pharmacology and Therapeutics* **43:** 542–546.

Coriat P, Richer C, Douraki T et al (1994) Influence of chronic angiotensin-converting enzyme inhibition on anesthetic induction. *Anesthesiology* **81:** 299–307.

Davies T, Lederer DA, Spencer AA & McNicol GP (1974) The effects of flurbiprofen on platelet function and blood coagulation. *Thombosis Research* **5:** 667–683.

Digitalis Investigation Group (1997) The effect of digoxin on mortality and morbidity in patients with heart failure. *New England Journal of Medicine* **336:** 525–533.

Europe Research Group (1997) Perioperative sympatholysis. *Anesthesiology* **86:** 346–363.

Fauno P, Petersen KD & Husted SE (1993) Increased blood loss after preoperative NSAID. A retrospective study of 186 hip arthroplasties. *Acta Orthopaedica Scandinavica* **64:** 522–524.

Ferraris VA & Swanson E (1983) Aspirin usage and perioperative blood loss in patients undergoing unexpected operations. *Surgery, Gynecology and Obstetrics* **156:** 439–442.

Flacke JW, Bloor BC, Flacke WE et al (1987) Reduced narcotic requirements by clonidine with improved hemodynamic and adrenergic stability in patients undergoing coronary bypass surgery. *Anesthesiology* **67:** 11–19.

Furberg CD, Psaty BM & Meyer JV (1995) Nifedipine—dose related increase in mortality in patients with coronary artery disease. *Circulation* **92:** 1326–1331.

Gallagher JD, Gessman LJ, Nowa P & Kerns D (1986) Electrophysiologic effects of halothane and quinidine on canine cardiac Purkinje fibers: evidence for a synergic interaction. *Anesthesiology* **65:** 278–285.

Gavras H (1990) Angiotensin converting enzyme inhibition and its impact on cardiovascular disease. *Circulation* **81:** 381–388.

Henry PD (1980) Comparative pharmacology of calcium antagonists: nifedipine, verapamil and diltiazem. *American Journal of Cardiology* **46:** 1047–1057.

Jensen K, Bunemann L, Riisager S & Thomsen LJ (1989) Cerebral blood flow during anaesthesia: influence of pretreatment with metoprolol or captopril. *British Journal of Anaesthesia* **62:** 321–323.

Kapur PA, Bloor BC, Flacke WE & Olewine SK (1984a) Comparison of cardiovascular responses to verapamil during enflurane, isoflurane or halothane anesthesia in the dog. *Anesthesiology* **61:** 156–160.

Kapur PA, Norel EJ, Cowen GR & Dajee M (1984b) Verapamil administration after high doses of fentanyl with or without chronic nifedipine therapy in man. *Anesthesia and Analgesia* **63:** 231.

Kataja JHK, Kaukinen S, Viinimaki OVK et al (1989) Hemodynamic and hormonal changes in patients pretreated with captopril for surgery of the abdominal aorta. *Journal of Cardiothoracic Anesthesia* **3:** 425–432.

Kiowski W, Erne P, Bertel O et al (1986) Acute and chronic sympathetic reflex activation and anti-hypertensive response to nifedipine. Reports on hypertension. *Journal of the American College of Cardiology* **7:** 344–348.

Licker M, Neidhart P, Lustenberger S et al (1996) Long-term angiotensin-converting enzyme inhibitor treatment attenuates adrenergic responsiveness without altering hemodynamic control in patients undergoing cardiac surgery. *Anesthesiology* **84:** 789–800.

Mangano DT, Layug EL, Wallace A & Tateo I (1996) Effect of atenolol on mortality and cardiovascular morbidity after non cardiac surgery. *New England Journal of Medicine* **335:** 1713–1720.

Miller ED, Ackerly JA & Peach MJ (1978a) Blood pressure support during general anesthesia in a renin-dependent state in the rat. *Anesthesiology* **48:** 404–408.

Miller ED, Longnecker DE & Peach MJ (1978b) The regulatory function of the renin–angiotensin system during general anesthesia. *Anesthesiology* **48:** 399–403.

Mirenda JV & Grissom TE (1991) Anesthetic implications of the renin–angiotensin system and angiotensin-converting enzyme inhibitors. *Anesthesia and Analgesia* **72:** 667–683.

Muzi M, Goff DR, Kampine JP et al (1992) Clonidine reduces sympathetic activation but maintains baroreflex responses in normotensive humans. *Anesthesiology* **77:** 864–871.

O'Kelly B, Browner WS, Massie B et al (1992) The Study of Perioperative Ischemia Research Group. Ventricular arrhythmias in patients undergoing noncardiac surgery. *Journal of the American Medical Association* **268:** 217–221.

Packer M, Gheorghiade M, Young JB et al (1993) Withdrawal of digoxin from patients with chronic heart failure treated with angiotensin converting enzyme inhibitors. *New England Journal of Medicine* **329:** 1–7.

Pflugfelder PW, Baird MG, Tonkon MJ et al (1995) Clinical consequences of angiotensin-converting enzyme inhibitor withdrawal in chronic heart failure: a double-blind, placebo-controlled study of quinapril. The Quinapril Heart Failure Trial investigators. *Journal of the American College of Cardiology* **22(6):** 1557–1563.

Quintin L, Bonnet F, Macquin I et al (1990) Aortic surgery: effect of clonidine on intraoperative catecholaminergic and circulatory stability. *Acta Anaesthesiologica Scandinavica* **34:** 132–137.

Quintin L, Viale JP, Annat G et al (1991) Oxygen uptake after major abdominal surgery: effect of clonidine. *Anesthesiology* **74:** 236–241.

Quintin L, Bouilloc X, Butin E et al (1996) Clonidine for major vascular surgery in hypertensive patients: a double-blind, controlled, randomized study. *Anesthesia and Analgesia* **83:** 687–695.

Rinkenberger RL, Preystowksy EN, Heger JJ et al (1980) Effects of intravenous and chronic and verapamil administration in patients with supraventricular tachyarrythmias. *Circulation* **62:** 996–1010.

Roizen MF (1988) Should we all have a sympathectomy at birth? Or at least preoperatively? *Anesthesiology* **68:** 482–484 (editorial).

Ryckwaert F & Colson P (1997) Hemodynamic effects of anesthesia in patients with ischemic heart failure chronically treated with angiotensin converting enzyme inhibitors. *Anesthesia and Analgesia* **84:** 945–949.

SOLVD Investigators (1991) Effect of enalapril on survival in patients with reduced left ventricular ejection fraction and congestive heart failure. *New England Journal of Medicine* **325:** 293–301.

Still JC, Nugent M, Moyer TP et al (1985) Plasma levels of beta-blocking drugs prior to coronary artery bypass surgery. *Anesthesiology* **62:** 67–70.

Stone JG, Foex P, Sear JW et al (1988) Myocardial ischemia in untreated hypertensive patients: effect of a single small oral dose of a β-adrenergic blocking agent. *Anesthesiology* **68:** 495–500.

Todd PA & Heel RC (1986) Enalapril: a review of its pharmacodynamic and pharmacokinetic properties, and therapeutic use in hypertension and congestive heart failure. *Drugs* **31:** 198–248.

Vidt DG, Bravo EL & Fouad FM (1982) Captopril. *New England Journal of Medicine* **306:** 214–219.

Wallace A, Layug B, Tateo I et al (1998) Prophylactic atenolol reduces postoperative myocardial ischemia. *Anesthesiology* **88:** 7–17.

Waltier DC (1998) Beta-adrenergic-blocking drugs: incredibly useful, incredibly underutilized. *Anesthesiology* **88:** 2–5.

Williams JF, Bristow MR, Fowler MB et al (1995) Guidelines for the evaluation and management of heart failure. *Circulation* **92:** 2764–2784.

Woosley RL (1991) Antiarrhythmic drugs. *Annual Review of Pharmacology and Toxicology* **31:** 427–455.

# 7

# Pre-operative cardiac interventions in non-cardiac surgery

HELFRIED METZLER MD

Professor of Anaesthesiology

*Department of Anaesthesiology and Intensive Care Medicine, University of Graz, Auenbruggerplatz 29, A-8036 Graz, Austria*

LEE A. FLEISHER MD

Associate Professor of Anesthesiology and Critical Care Medicine, Joint Appointment in Medicine (Cardiology) and Health Policy and Management

*Johns Hopkins Medical Institutions, Carnegie 442, 600 North Wolfe Street, Baltimore, Maryland 21287, USA*

Pre-operative cardiac interventions may be performed before a planned non-cardiac surgical procedure in order to optimize the patient's status and to reduce peri-operative morbidity and mortality (MM). The interventional procedures in patients with coronary artery disease are coronary artery bypass graft surgery and percutaneous transluminal coronary angioplasty, in patients with severe aortic stenosis, aortic valve replacement or aortic balloon valvuloplasty. These procedures can only be recommended if surgery without intervention would result in a higher peri-operative MM than the direct approach. Several aspects make the decision process difficult: lack of prospective randomized trials, specific indications for specific procedures, small cohorts of clinical studies, changing management in surgery, anaesthesiology and cardiology, and the influence on short- and long-term outcome. Excellent decision analysis models and guidelines of task forces, however, may help the clinician to obtain sufficient support for his or her pre-operative strategies. Finally, the local experience of the surgical, anaesthesiological and cardiological team has to be taken into consideration before the decision is made, if the individual patient is to benefit from the pre-operative interventional procedure.

**Key words:** coronary artery disease; aortic stenosis; coronary artery bypass graft surgery; percutaneous transluminal angioplasty; aortic valve replacement; balloon valvuloplasty; peri-operative morbidity and mortality.

*Baillière's Clinical Anaesthesiology—*
Vol. 12, No. 3, September 1998
ISBN 0–7020–2536–4
0950–3501/98/030419 + 14 $12.00/00

# CORONARY ARTERY DISEASE: CORONARY ARTERY BYPASS GRAFT SURGERY AND PERCUTANEOUS TRANSLUMINAL CORONARY ANGIOPLASTY

## Introduction

Several management strategies may be used in patients with coronary artery disease (CAD) presenting for non-cardiac surgery: immediate clearance, medical pre-treatment, interventional procedures, delay or cancellation (Figure 1). Pre-operative interventional procedures are only justified or may be recommended if the overall benefit outweighs the risk. The overall risk of a pre-operative intervention strategy includes morbidity and mortality resulting from invasive pre-operative testing, the interventional procedure, the delay of non-cardiac surgery and complications of the non-cardiac surgical procedure per se (Figure 2).

Additionally, when looking at the risk–benefit of any pre-operative procedure it is necessary to consider not only acute peri-operative morbidity and mortality but also long-term outcome.

In the following chapter technique, indications and risk of CABG surgery will briefly be compared with the interventional catheterization techniques including PTCA and stents.

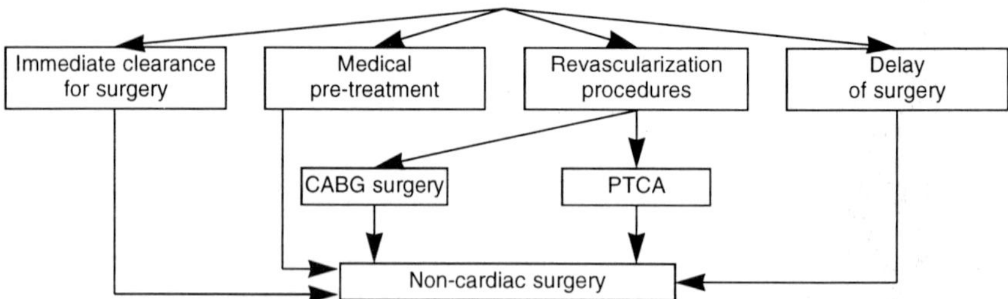


**Figure 1.** Preoperative management strategies in CAD patients before non-cardiac surgery (CABG, coronary artery bypass graft; PTCA, percutaneous transluminal angioplasty).

| $MM_a$ | $>$ | $MM_{b+c+d+e}$ |
|---|---|---|
| MM | | Morbidity and mortality resulting from |
| a | | Non-cardiac surgery without intervention |
| b | | Pre-operative extensive testing |
| c | | Pre-operative revascularization procedure |
| d | | Delay of non-cardiac surgery |
| e | | Non-cardiac surgery after intervention |

**Figure 2.** A net benefit of pre-operative interventions only exists if $MM_a > MM_{b+c+d+e}$.

## Percutaneous transluminal coronary angioplasty

A balloon angioplasty catheter is advanced via the femoral artery under local anaesthesia to the stenotic area in the coronary artery and is then inflated over a period of seconds or minutes. Indications are listed in special guidelines (Ryan et al, 1993). In this chapter the indications for the non-cardiac surgical patient are summarized (Ryan et al, 1993).

### *Single-vessel coronary artery disease*

*Class I indications.* This category applies to patients who have a significant lesion in a major epicardial artery that subtends a large area of viable myocardium and who must undergo high-risk non-cardiac surgery, if angina is present or there is objective evidence of ischaemia.

### *Multivessel coronary artery disease*

*Class I indications.* This category applies to patients who have one significant lesion in a major epicardial artery that could result in nearly complete revascularization because the additional lesion(s) subtend(s) a small viable or non-viable area of myocardium and who are undergoing high-risk non-cardiac surgery and demonstrate objective evidence of myocardial ischaemia.

### *Procedural complications* (Lincoff and Topol, 1997)

The reported incidence of myocardial infarction (MI) after PTCA is 1.0% and the in-hospital mortality 4.3%. The current emergency bypass rate is about 0.9% (2–5%). The most critical complication associated with PTCA is the abrupt vessel closure with an incidence of 3–8%.

### *The problem of inadequate prediction of the site of a peri-operative myocardial infarction*

Any pre-operative strategy to perform PTCA in a patient with a significant stenosis follows the rationale that peri-operative MIs occur most probably at the site of the most significant lesion. Little et al (1988) have shown that the angiographic severity of coronary artery stenosis in cardiological patients must not necessarily predict the time or location of a subsequent coronary occlusion. In a recent paper Dawood et al (1996) confirmed these findings also for peri-operative MIs. In their study, predicting the site of MI based on severity of underlying stenosis would have been unsuccessful in more than half of the patients (Dawood et al, 1996). Ellis et al (1996) found that the most common cause of infarction in CAD patients undergoing major non-thoracic vascular surgery was collateral vessels inadequate to prevent MI during the stress of surgery. High-grade stenoses (>70%) were an uncommon cause of complications (Ellis et al, 1996). All these studies may help to explain some of the relatively disappointing results of PTCA in the peri-operative setting.

If non-cardiac surgery is planned after PTCA there should be an interval of several days before surgery because of the need for coronary plaque and/or myocardial stabilization. However, it should be performed in <1–2 months due to the risk of restenosis (Eagle et al, 1996).

## Intracoronary stents

Coronary artery stenting is a novel treatment for coronary stenosis (Lincoff and Topol, 1997; Versaci et al, 1997). Intracoronary stents are tubes, currently composed of various metals, which are able to support and to stretch a diseased segment of coronary artery. The advantages of stenting compared with standard PTCA are under investigation, especially the advantage of a lower restenosis rate (Lincoff and Topol, 1997; Versaci et al, 1997). The major disadvantage of stents in clinical use results from their potential of thrombogenicity (Lincoff and Topol, 1997). Anecdotal reports of acute thrombotic closure, distal embolization or bleeding from intensive anti-coagulation suggest that at the moment this new technique should not be used in the peri-operative scenario.

## Coronary artery bypass graft surgery

For years saphenous veins were used for surgical revascularization under cardiopulmonary bypass. In the meantime the internal mammary artery (IMA) is used more frequently, and recently CABG surgery without cardiopulmonary bypass and a small approach without sternotomy (minimal invasive CABG surgery) is becoming more popular. When these techniques are established they should result in a better outcome and a shorter hospital stay.

### *Indications* (American College of Cardiology–American Heart Association, 1991; Eagle et al, 1996)

In patients whose angina is not controlled by medical management and who are, on the basis of their coronary anatomy not candidates for PTCA, CABG surgery is indicated. The highest benefit of CABG surgery is well documented for patients with multivessel disease and left ventricular (LV) dysfunction, irrespective of symptoms. In patients whose dominant symptom is heart failure without severe angina, the benefit of coronary revascularization is less well defined.

### *Procedural complications* (Gersh and Braunwald, 1997)

The reported overall mortality of elective CABG surgery ranges from 1.3% to 2.6% depending on the use of IMA grafts. The benefit of newer techniques will probably be antagonized by the shift towards multimorbid older patients.

## Angiography

The first step in any pre-operative interventional procedure has to be made by the decision of invasive pre-operative testing. Coronary arteriography is the imaging method of choice for the diagnosis of CAD and for deciding on further strategies: medical treatment, PTCA or bypass surgery. The complication rate with the femoral approach is low, with a mortality of 0.1%. Non-fatal MI occurs in 0.07%, neurological complications occur in 0.14% and vascular complications in 0.35% (Lincoff and Topol, 1997)

## Available clinical studies

The 'ignition' paper about the fundamental question of the benefit of pre-operative revascularization was published in 1984 by the group of N. R. Hertzer of the Cleveland Clinic Foundation (Hertzer et al, 1984). Papers before that time should not be taken into consideration, because there has been a dramatic change in surgical, cardiological and anaesthetic management, so that these data do not allow a valid conclusion. Hertzer et al were the first group to demonstrate that patients with severe, but surgically correctable, CAD, who were advised to undergo myocardial revascularization preceding vascular surgery, might benefit from CABG surgery. They observed an early mortality of 2% but only of 0.8% in the group having previous CABG surgery. The overall operative mortality for CABG and vascular procedures was 2.6%.

In the following years several studies addressed the same question looking at both CABG surgery and PTCA (Foster et al, 1986; Golden et al, 1990; Allen et al, 1991; Gottlieb, 1991; Huber et al, 1992; Lachapelle et al, 1992; Nielsen et al, 1992; Elmore et al, 1993; Zubicki et al, 1995; Eagle et al, 1997; Fleisher et al, 1997). The studies are listed in Table 1. Most of them analysed the data retrospectively; no large prospective studies are available. Recently Eagle et al (1997) analysed the patient population of the Coronary Artery Surgery Study (CASS) registry. They found that vascular, thoracic, abdominal and major head and neck surgeries were associated with a higher risk of MI or death in the face of a non-revascularized CAD. Patients with advanced angina, patients over 60 years of age and patients with multivessel disease will benefit the most. Coronary revascularization protected from peri-operative MI for at least 6 years after revascularization.

A limited amount of data addressed the question of pre-operative PTCA versus CABG surgery, allowing no interpretation, because PTCA is indicated in a selective subgroup of patients. In non-surgical CAD patients, PTCA and CABG have their specific indications and both techniques as well as medical therapy should not be seen as competitive but rather complementary strategies (Pocock et al, 1995; Bypass Angioplasty Revascularization Investigation Investigators, 1996; Hlatky et al, 1997; Jackson, 1997).

Fleisher et al (1997) used a 5% sample of the medicare database for 6

**Table 1.** Outcome studies about cardiac interventions before non-cardiac surgery.

| Reference | Design | Type of surgery | Intervention |
|---|---|---|---|
| Hertzer et al (1984) | Prospective | VS | CABG |
| Foster et al (1986) | Retrospective | VS | CABG |
| Golden et al (1990) | Retrospective | VS | CABG |
| Allen et al (1991) | Retrospective | VS + NVS | CABG–PTCA |
| Gottlieb (1991) | Retrospective | VS | PTCA |
| Huber et al (1992) | Retrospective | VS + NVS | PTCA |
| Lachapelle et al (1992) | Retrospective | VS | CABG |
| Nielsen et al (1992) | Retrospective | VS + NVS | CABG |
| Elmore et al (1993) | Retrospective | VS | CABG–PTCA |
| Zubicki et al (1995) | Retrospective | VS | PTCA |
| Fleisher et al (1997) | Retrospective | VS | CABG–PTCA |
| Eagle et al (1997) | Retrospective | VS | CABG |

VS, vascular surgery; NVS, non-vascular surgery.

months of 1991. A high incidence of peri-operative and long-term morbidity and mortality in patients who had not undergone pre-operative testing was found. Amazingly, pre-operative PTCA was associated with a relatively high peri-operative and long-term mortality suggesting the need for re-evaluation of PTCA in this setting.

## Decision analysis models

From the available clinical studies, although they provide a broad spectrum of information, no clear recommendations based on hard data can be given. Therefore, two groups used decision analysis models trying to justify each step of pre-operative assessment and intervention in a decision process and to assign probability for each potential outcome (Fleisher et al, 1994; Mason et al, 1995). From the available data decision trees were constructed. Fleisher et al (1994) looked at coronary artery revascularization before abdominal aortic aneurysm surgery, which represents one of the non-cardiac surgical procedures with the highest risk. In their two-way sensitivity analysis of mortality, pre-operative testing and subsequent coronary revascularization seems to be the preferred option for most typical values in a patient with a high prior probability of CAD, whereas, in patients with a very low prior probability of CAD, surgery alone seems to be the preferred option (Figure 3). Fleisher et al also demonstrated that the optimal pre-operative strategy depends on local factors.

The objective of Mason et al's (1995) decision analysis was to determine short-term outcome in patients presenting for non-cardiac vascular surgery with and without pre-operative angiography plus revascularization. Proceeding directly to vascular surgery led to decreased mortality and cost in the base case analysis. The angiography strategy led to higher mortality if vascular surgery proceeded in patients with inoperable CAD but led to slightly lower mortality if vascular surgery was cancelled in patients with inoperable CAD. The coronary angiography strategy also led to lower mortality when vascular surgery was particularly risky.

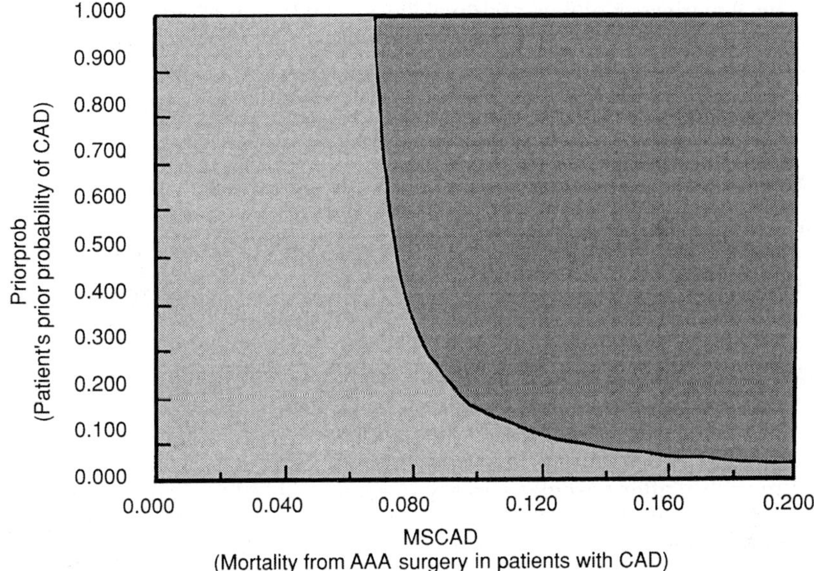


**Figure 3.** A two-way sensitivity analysis demonstrating the optimal pre-operative strategy of surgery alone or coronary revascularization before vascular surgery: ▒, surgery; ▓, test. As the probability of mortality from coronary revascularization increases, then vascular surgery alone is the preferred strategy. In contrast, as the probability of mortality from aortic surgery in patients with significant CAD increases, then coronary revascularization before vascular surgery is the optimal strategy. The average mortality for vascular surgery in patients with significant CAD is 9.5%, suggesting that the strategy with the lowest mortality is very sensitive to local morbidity and mortality. However, if long-term mortality is included in the model, the coronary revascularization might prove to be more beneficial. Reproduced from Fleisher et al (1994, *Anesthesia and Analgesia* **79:** 661–669) with permission.

## Guidelines of task forces

The American College of Cardiology (ACC) – American Heart Association (AHA) Task Force for pre-operative evaluation published an excellent, detailed review on the rationale for surgical coronary revascularization and PTCA (Eagle et al, 1996). They stated that no good randomized trials have assessed the benefit of prophylactic CABG surgery and that the number of retrospective studies demonstrated a lower peri-operative mortality rate in association with non-cardiac procedures. The decision to perform revascularization in a patient before non-cardiac surgery may only be recommended in a small subset of very high-risk patients.

Patients undergoing elective non-cardiac procedures, who are found to have prognostic high-risk coronary anatomy and in whom long-term outcome would be likely to be improved by CABG surgery, should generally undergo revascularization before an elective surgical procedure of high or intermediate risk. For PTCA the Task Force stated that the role of this technique is currently incompletely defined and that indications for PTCA in the peri-operative setting are identical to those published by the ACC–AHA Task Force for the use of PTCA in general.

The American College of Physicians (1997) published guidelines for pre-operative management of CAD patients. Their recommendations are also based on the previously mentioned task force reports and decision analysis models.

## Short- and long-term outcome of pre-operative revascularization

The anaesthesiologist's role in peri-operative care implies his or her main interest in reducing peri-operative cardiac complications. The option of pre-operative interventional procedures is therefore mainly assessed with respect to lowering the peri-operative risk. Any 'prophylactic' pre-operative revascularization procedure, however, has to be viewed, independently of the upcoming surgical procedure, for its effect not only on the short- but also on the long-term outcome, which may have a substantial influence on quality of life and cost (Fleisher et al, 1994).

Coronary events are the most important causes of long-term morbidity and mortality after vascular surgery (Criqui et al, 1992; Rihal et al, 1992, 1995; Farouk et al, 1994). On the basis of CASS data Rihal et al (1995) concluded that the long-term outcome among patients with CAD and peripheral vascular disease was improved by revascularization, and the beneficial effects were not offset by the initial higher risk for patients undergoing CABG surgery. Therefore, in the final decision of 'prophylactic' pre-operative revascularization the urgency of the non-cardiac surgical procedure, the severity of the CAD, the likelihood of a successful procedure, the age of the patient and the influence of such an intervention on the long-term outcome have to be judged by the team who takes care of the patient.

## Conclusions

Summarizing the results of available clinical studies, the findings of decision analysis models and the comment of task forces, the following recommendations can be given.

1. Clinically stable patients undergoing low- and intermediate-risk procedures will not benefit from extensive pre-operative testing and revascularization procedures.
2. A potential benefit only exists for patients with severe CAD if these patients undergo high-risk procedures and if there is a high likelihood of successful revascularization.
3. Currently, indications for pre-operative CABG and PTCA do not differ from those given for non-surgical patients.
4. Currently, coronary stent placement cannot be recommended for use in the peri-operative setting.
5. Finally, local specific factors including experience in different techniques and outcome-oriented quality of work of the cardiological, surgical and anaesthesiological team contribute to the decision in an individual centre.

## VALVULAR HEART DISEASE: VALVE REPLACEMENT AND BALLOON VALVULOPLASTY

### Introduction

Severe valvular disease in patients presenting for non-cardiac surgery is a major clinical predictor of increased peri-operative cardiovascular risk, necessitating careful pre-operative assessment and management, which may result in delay, cancellation of or pre-operative intervention before surgery unless it is an emergency (Goldman, 1987; Eagle et al, 1996).

Symptomatic stenotic lesions (aortic and mitral valve stenosis) are associated with a higher risk of peri-operative complications than symptomatic regurgitations (aortic and mitral valve insufficiency), which are usually better tolerated in the peri-operative setting or may also be stabilized pre-operatively with medical pre-treatment (Eagle et al, 1996).

Severe aortic stenosis is the valvular disease with the highest risk for non-cardiac surgical patients and will therefore be discussed in the following section.

### Assessment of aortic stenosis

*Pre-operative evaluation*

In contrast to mitral stenosis a long latent period exists with increasing obstruction of and pressure load on the LV myocardium while the patient remains asymptomatic. Main clinical manifestations are angina pectoris, syncope and heart failure. Once these symptoms become manifest and are not treated adequately the prognosis is poor. A typical example of a patient who presents to the anaesthesiologist pre-operatively is the 75 year old patient with hip fracture after an unexplained fall (syncope). Complete pre-operative assessment includes an electrocardiogram (ECG), chest X-ray, echocardiography and/or angiography.

*Classification of the severity of aortic stenosis* (Braunwald, 1997)

Critical obstruction to left ventricular outflow is generally considered if

- effective aortic orifice in an average-sized adult is $<0.8\,cm^2$, or $<0.5\,cm^2/m^2$ body surface area (BSA) or
- peak systolic pressure difference exceeds 50 mmHg in the presence of a normal cardiac output.

*Pre-operative decision process*

Optional pre-operative management includes

- medical pre-treatment (recompensation, etc.),
- open surgical repair before non-cardiac surgery,

- balloon valvuloplasty before non-cardiac surgery,
- clearance for surgery without further pre-operative intervention and
- cancellation of surgery.

**Aortic valve replacement** (Atkins et al, 1997; Braunwald, 1997; Connolly et al, 1997; Bernal et al, 1998)

Indications for aortic valve replacement are symptomatic patients with haemodynamic evidence of severe obstruction as well as asymptomatic patients with progressive LV dysfunction and/or significant ventricular ectopic activity. Mortality ranges from 2% to 9% in most centres and may decrease to 1% in patients under the age of 70 years. Poor LV function, concomitant CAD and age are significantly correlated with increased per-operative mortality. In patients with concomitant CAD, a relatively common combination, aortic valve replacement can and should be performed together with myocardial revascularization.

### Balloon aortic valvuloplasty

Indications in non-surgical patients are cardiogenic shock, advanced age, and bridging to valve replacement in patients with severe heart failure who are at extremely high operative risk, in pregnant women with critical stenosis and in patients who refuse surgical pre-treatment (Braunwald, 1997).

The mortality of the procedure is about 3% and 30 day mortality 14%. Restenosis occurs early and long-term survival is poor (Otto et al, 1994).

In surgical patients balloon valvuloplasty may be performed if the patients are not candidates for valve surgery and if non-cardiac surgery is elective or in patients with semi-elective non-cardiac surgical procedures. These patients may benefit from balloon valvuloplasty, because the non-cardiac surgical procedure may be performed within 24 hours of the balloon valvuloplasty and there is sudden relief of extreme stenosis. Restenosis occurring after months does not play a significant role in the immediate post-operative period.

In 1988 and 1989 two groups published their first reports on palliative percutaneous aortic balloon valvuloplasty before non-cardiac operations (Levine et al, 1988; Hayes et al, 1989). Levine et al reported data on seven patients and Hayes et al on nine patients. In both groups the procedure was performed without complications as well as subsequent non-cardiac surgery. Recently, the procedure was re-evaluated by Weihs et al (1996). They reported on eight patients with severe aortic stenosis (aortic valve area (AVA) $0.5 \pm 0.1$ cm$^2$/m$^2$ BSA) and poor LV function (ejection fraction $29 \pm 7$%). The procedure was successful in all patients (AVA $0.8 \pm 1$ cm$^2$/m$^2$, mean difference $29 \pm 15$ mmHg). After the procedure one patient with congestive heart failure died before non-cardiac surgery; all other patients underwent non-cardiac surgery within 48 hours of the valvuloplasty without peri-operative cardiac complications.

## Clearance for surgery without any pre-operative intervention

In the last two decades peri-operative anaesthesiological management has dramatically improved: new pharmacological and monitoring strategies offer instruments for the anaesthesiologist to avoid haemodynamic catastrophes in severe aortic stenosis or to treat them adequately. The first retrospective study looking at the risk of non-cardiac surgery in a selected group of patients with severe aortic stenosis was published in 1989 (O'Keefe et al, 1989). Recently, two studies published data on patients with severe aortic stenosis undergoing non-cardiac surgery without further pre-operative intervention (Tang et al, 1998; Torsher et al, 1998). In one study 19 patients underwent 28 surgical procedures, 26 performed under general and two under spinal anaesthesia. Intraoperatively, one patient required temporary pacing and two patients died post-operatively owing to peri-operative MI and multiple organ failure (Torsher et al, 1998). Tang et al (1998) reported on 40 patients undergoing 42 procedures. They included patients with an AVA $\leq 1\ cm^2$ or a peak gradient >60 mmHg. Mortality was 1.9%; the most common peri-operative complication was post-operative pulmonary oedema while congestive heart failure occurred in 17.3% and MI in 1.3%.

## Cancellation of surgery

Depending on the age of the patient, the general status and the necessity for the surgical procedure, the responsible team including the surgeon, cardiologist and anaesthesiologist should define a benefit:risk ratio of the planned procedure and discuss the problem with the patient and may conclude in some rare cases to cancel surgery altogether.

## Pre-operative decision process

Currently, clear recommendations do not exist for the final decision, whether and which pre-operative intervention for an individual patient may be preferable. Existing data do not support a certain approach, no prospective studies outweight one strategy against the other and the number of patients in the cohorts are too small to give them sufficient statistical power.

A feasible pre-operative algorithm is depicted in Figure 4.

In patients awaiting elective non-cardiac surgery with expected high risk according to cardiac risk stratification, pre-operative aortic valve replacement still seems to remain the primary treatment.

If the patient is not a candidate for non-cardiac surgery, the non-cardiac surgical procedure is semi-elective and the institution performing interventional cardiology including balloon valvuloplasty has a great deal of experience with this procedure, balloon valvuloplasty may be undertaken, giving the chance to perform non-cardiac surgery within 48 hours after the intervention.

Finally, non-cardiac surgery may be performed with an experienced anaesthesiological and surgical team without further pre-operative inter-

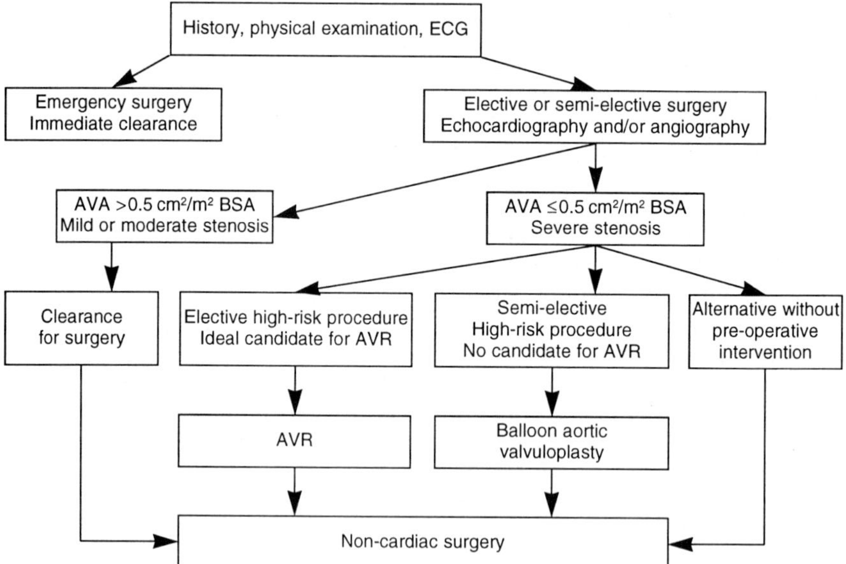


**Figure 4.** Decision tree in patients with suspected aortic stenosis (AVR, aortic valve replacement).

vention with an acceptable risk. On the basis of our current knowledge of peri-operative pathophysiology, it becomes increasingly clear, however, that also for the patient with severe aortic stenosis it is not the intra-operative period with the option to use all the advantages of new anaesthetic drugs and monitoring devices that brings about the risk of complications but the immediate post-operative period with the imposed haemodynamic stress on the left ventricle.

## ADDENDUM

Recently, new guidelines for the management of patients with valvular heart disease have been published by the American College of Cardiology and the American Heart Association, also addressing the management of patients with severe aortic stenosis (American College of Cardiology and American Heart Association, 1998).

## REFERENCES

Allen JR, Helling TS & Hartzler GO (1991) Operative procedures not involving the heart after percutaneous transluminal coronary angioplasty. *Surgery, Gynecology and Obstetrics* **173:** 285–288.

American College of Cardiology–American Heart Association (1991) ACC/AHA guidelines and indications for coronary artery bypass graft surgery. A report of the American College of

Cardiology–American Heart Association Task Force on Assessment of Diagnostic and Therapeutic Cardiovascular Procedures (Subcommittee on Coronary Artery Bypass Graft Surgery). *Circulation* **83:** 1125–1173.

American College of Cardiology–American Heart Association (1998) ACC/AHA guidelines for the management of patients with valvular heart disease (Committee on Management of Patients with Valvular Heart Disease). *Circulation* **98:** 1949–1984.

*American College of Physicians (1997) Guidelines for assessing and managing the perioperative risk from coronary artery disease associated with major noncardiac surgery. *Annals of Internal Medicine* **127:** 309–312.

Atkins CW, Daggett WM, Vlahakes GJ et al (1997) Cardiac operations in patients 80 years old and older. *Annals of Thoracic Surgery* **64:** 606–614.

Bernal JM, Rabasa JM, Gutierrez GF et al (1988) The CarboMedics valve: experience with 1,049 implants. *Annals of Thoracic Surgery* **65:** 137–143.

*Braunwald E (1997) Valvular heart disease. In Braunwald E (ed.) *Heart Disease*, pp 1007–1076. Philadelphia, PA: WB Saunders.

*Bypass Angioplasty Revascularization Investigation Investigators (1996) Comparison of coronary bypass surgery with angioplasty in patients with multivessel disease. *New England Journal of Medicine* **335:** 217–225.

Connolly HM, Oh JK, Orszulak TA et al (1997) Aortic valve replacement for aortic stenosis with severe left ventricular dysfunction. Prognostic indicators. *Circulation* **95:** 2395–2400.

Criqui MH, Langer RD, Fronek A et al (1992) Mortality over a period of 10 years in patients with peripheral arterial disease. *New England Journal of Medicine* **326:** 381–386.

Dawood MM, Gutpa DK, Southern J et al (1996) Pathology of fatal perioperative myocardial infarction: implications regarding pathophysiology and prevention. *International Journal of Cardiology* **57:** 37–44.

*Eagle KA, Brundage BH, Chaitman et al (1996) Guidelines for perioperative cardiovascular evaluation for noncardiac surgery. Report of the American College of Cardiology/American Heart Association Task Force on Practice Guidelines. *Circulation* **93:** 1278–1317.

*Eagle KA, Rihal CS, Mickel MC et al (1997) Cardiac risk of noncardiac surgery: influence of coronary disease and type of surgery in 3368 operations. CASS Investigators and University of Michigan Heart Care Program. Coronary Artery Surgery Study. *Circulation* **96:** 1882–1887.

Ellis SG, Hertzer NR, Young JR & Brener S (1996) Angiographic correlates of cardiac death and myocardial infarction complicating major nonthoracic vascular surgery. *American Journal of Cardiology* **77:** 1126–1128.

Elmore JR, Hallett JWJ, Gibbons RJ et al (1993) Myocardial revascularization before abdominal aortic aneurysmorrhaphy: effect of coronary angioplasty. *Mayo Clinic Proceedings* **68:** 637–641.

Farouk MD, Rihal CS, Gersh BJ et al (1994) Influence of coronary heart disease on morbidity and mortality after lower extremity revascularization surgery: a population-based study in Olmsted County, Minnesota. *Journal of the American College of Cardiology* **24:** 1290–1296.

*Fleisher LA, Skolnick ED, Holroyd KJ & Lehmann HP (1994) Coronary artery revascularization before abdominal aortic aneurysm surgery: a decision analytic approach. *Anesthesia and Analgesia* **79:** 661–669.

Fleisher LA, Eagle KA, Shaffer T & Anderson G (1997) Mortality after major vascular surgery: analysis of the medicare database. *Anesthesia and Analgesia* **84:** SAC43.

Foster ED, Davis KB, Carpenter JA et al (1986) Risk of noncardiac operation in patients with defined coronary disease: the Coronary Artery Surgery Study (CASS) registry experience. *Annals of Thoracic Surgery* **41:** 42–50.

Gersh BJ & Braunwald E (1997) Chronic coronary artery disease. In Braunwald E (ed.) *Heart Disease*, pp 1289–1365. Philadelphia, PA: WB Saunders.

Golden MA, Whittemore AD, Donaldson MC & Mannick JA (1990) Selective evaluation and management of coronary artery disease in patients undergoing repair of abdominal aortic aneurysms. A 16-year experience. *Annals of Surgery* **212:** 415–420.

Goldman L (1987) Multifactorial index of cardiac risk in noncardiac surgery: ten-year status report. *Journal of Cardiothoracic Anesthesia* **1:** 237–244.

Gottlieb A (1991) The incidence of perioperative myocardial infarction (PMI) in patients with prior percutaneous transluminal coronary angioplasty (PTCA). *Anesthesiology* **75:** A52.

Hayes SN, Holmes DR Jr, Nishimura RA & Reeder GS (1989) Palliative percutaneous aortic balloon valvuloplasty before noncardiac operations and invasive diagnostic procedures. *Mayo Clinic Proceedings* **64:** 753–757.

Hertzer NR, Beven EG, Young JR et al (1984) Coronary artery disease in peripheral vascular patients. A classification of 1000 coronary angiograms and results of surgical management. *Annals of Surgery* **199:** 223–233.

Hlatky MA, Rogers WJ, Johnstone I et al (1997) Medical care costs and quality of life after randomization to coronary angioplasty or coronary bypass surgery. Bypass Angioplasty Revascularization Investigation (BARI) investigators. *New England Journal of Medicine* **336:** 92–99.

Huber KC, Evans MA, Bresnahan JF et al (1992) Outcome of noncardiac operations in patients with severe coronary artery disease successfully treated preoperatively with coronary angioplasty. *Mayo Clinic Proceedings* **67:** 15–21.

Jackson G (1997) Stable angina: drugs, angioplasty or surgery? *European Heart Journal* **18 (supplement B):** B2–B10.

Lachapelle K, Graham AM & Symes JF (1992) Does the clinical evaluation of the cardiac status predict outcome in patients with abdominal aortic aneurysms? *Journal of Vascular Surgery* **15:** 964–970.

Levine MJ, Berman AD, Safian RD et al (1988) Palliation of valvular aortic stenosis by balloon valvuloplasty as preoperative preparation for noncardiac surgery. *American Journal of Cardiology* **62:** 1309–1310.

*Lincoff AM & Topol EJ (1997) Interventional catheterization techniques. In Braunwald E (ed.) *Heart Disease*, pp 1366–1378. Philadelphia, PA: WB Saunders.

Little WC, Constantinescu M, Applegate RJ et al (1988) Can coronary angiography predict the site of a subsequent myocardial infarction in patients with mild-to-moderate coronary artery disease? *Circulation* **78:** 1157–1166.

*Mason JJ, Owens DK, Harris RA et al (1995) The role of coronary angiography and coronary revascularization before noncardiac vascular surgery. *Journal of the American Medical Association* **273:** 1919–1925.

Nielsen JL, Page CP, Mann C et al (1992) Risk of major elective operation after myocardial revascularization. *American Journal of Surgery* **164:** 423–426.

O'Keefe JH Jr, Shub C & Rettke SR (1989) Risk of noncardiac surgical procedures in patients with aortic stenosis. *Mayo Clinic Proceedings* **64:** 400–405.

Otto CM, Mickel MC, Kennedy JW et al (1994) Three-year outcome after balloon aortic valvuloplasty. Insights into prognosis of valvular aortic stenosis. *Circulation* **89:** 642–650.

*Pocock SJ, Henderson RA, Rickards AF et al (1995) Meta-analysis of randomised trials comparing coronary angioplasty with bypass surgery. *Lancet* **346:** 1184–1189.

Rihal CS, Gersh BJ, Whisnant JP et al (1992) Influence of coronary heart disease on morbidity and mortality after carotid endarterectomy: a population-based study in Olmsted County, Minnesota (1970–1988). *Journal of the American College of Cardiology* **19:** 1254–1260.

Rihal CS, Eagle KA, Mickel MC et al (1995) Surgical therapy for coronary artery disease among patients with combined coronary artery and peripheral vascular disease. *Circulation* **91:** 46–53.

*Ryan TJ, Bauman WB, Kennedy JW et al (1993) Guidelines for percutaneous transluminal coronary angioplasty. A report of the American Heart Association/American College of Cardiology Task Force on Assessment of Diagnostic and Therapeutic Cardiovascular Procedures (Committee on Percutaneous Transluminal Coronary Angioplasty). *Circulation* **88:** 2987–3007.

Tang YS, Janelle GM, Lobato EB & Urdaneta F (1998) Aortic stenosis in patients undergoing noncardiac surgery: the University of Florida experience. *Anesthesia and Analgesia* **86:** SC113 (abstract).

Torsher LC, Shub C, Rettke SR & Brown DL (1998) Risk of patients with severe aortic stenosis undergoing noncardiac surgery. *American Journal of Cardiology* **81:** 448–452.

Versaci F, Gaspardone A, Tomai F et al (1997) A comparison of coronary-artery stenting with angioplasty for isolated stenosis of the proximal left anterior descending coronary artery. *New England Journal of Medicine* **336:** 817–822.

Weihs B, Metzler H, Prause G & List WF (1996) Preoperative aortic balloon valvuloplasty in patients with severe aortic stenosis and noncardiac surgery. *Acta Anaesthesiologia Scandinavica* **40 (supplement):** 256.

Zubicki A, Gosgnach ML, Bertrand M et al (1995) Long-term cardiac prognosis of percutaneous transluminal coronary angioplasty in patients with infrarenal aortic aneurysms. *British Journal of Anaesthesia* **74 (supplement):** 1.

# 8

# Pre-anaesthetic preparation of the emergency patient

ROBERT O. FENECK MB, BS, FRCA

Consultant Anaesthesiologist and Hon. Senior Lecturer
*St. Thomas's Hospital, Lambeth Palace Road, London SE1 7EH, UK*

Pre-anaesthetic preparation is a vital component of safe anaesthesia. The emergency patient is at higher risk in almost all surgical circumstances, not least because adequate preparation is more difficult. A variety of factors, including the nature of the emergency, cardiovascular disturbance, fluid shifts and the presence of a full stomach will render the patient more at risk. Furthermore, the presence of pre-existing disease, often poorly controlled, may further hazard the delivery of safe anaesthesia. This chapter explores these aspects in greater detail.

**Key words:** emergency; pre-medication; pre-anaesthetic preparation.

The use of the term 'emergency' has varied markedly. In the UK, the multidisciplinary team that set up the National Confidential Enquiry into Perioperative Deaths in 1988 defined an emergency as 'resuscitation simultaneous with surgical treatment. Operation usually within 1 hour'. More simply, the Working Party Report of the Royal College of Anaesthetists in 1996 defined an emergency 'as an operation on a patient not fully resuscitated', contrasting this with an urgent procedure described as 'an operation not on a routine operating list but in a patient fully resuscitated'. However we define it, it is clear that in the emergency patient there is a much smaller time frame for appropriate pre-operative investigation and work-up (Adams et al, 1998). Pre-anaesthetic preparation will have to be as good as possible in the time available and resuscitative treatment will be ongoing both during and probably after surgery. Pre-anaesthetic preparation will be influenced by a number of factors.

*Nature of the surgical emergency (e.g. trauma, major vascular, head and neck, obstetric)* There may be wide variation in cardiovascular stability, fluid and electrolyte status, conscious level, airway protection, blood gas homeostasis and the ability of the patient to self-ventilate, the presence of

*Baillière's Clinical Anaesthesiology—*
Vol. 12, No. 3, September 1998
ISBN 0–7020–2536–4
0950–3501/98/030433 + 18 $12.00/00

a full stomach and the dangers of aspiration, and a variety of other factors, many of which are dealt with below.

*Coexisting pathology* This may be related to the surgical condition under treatment or more frequently is independent of it. Anaesthesia at either extreme of age is identified as being at increased risk, and particularly so in the elderly where there is an increased risk of coexistent pathology including cardiovascular disease.

Furthermore, surgical emergencies may result in the loss of effective control of some conditions, including diabetes and hypertension, and some surgical emergencies are also more common in patients with diabetes. In other circumstances an acute medical condition may provoke an acute surgical emergency. For example, in patients with atrial fibrillation or following a recent myocardial infarction, a thrombus of cardiac origin may embolize the arterial tree causing a variety of surgical problems including an acute abdomen due to mesenteric embolus or a pulseless limb.

We should also recognize that there are certain categories of patients who present a risk of cross-infection to other patients and also to the medical and nursing staff. Where there are time or other constraints on testing for communicable diseases in high-risk patients (i.e. human immunodeficiency virus, hepatitis B and C) then the safe course of action is to assume that the patient represents an infective risk and to take appropriate measures to prevent cross-infection occurring.

The essential dilemma is that good preparation is the key to safe anaesthesia and surgery, but in the emergency patient time constraints may limit the effectiveness of preparation. No matter how critical the emergency, an appraisal of the state of the patient's airway with regard to the ease of endotracheal intubation and an assessment of the patient's circulation, fluid status and where appropriate electrolyte balance must be carried out.

## NATURE OF THE EMERGENCY

Some aspects of pre-anaesthetic preparation are common to all patients undergoing emergency surgery. These are considered below.

### Full stomach

The volume of gastric contents may be very variable. Many emergency patients will have taken food and drink recently before surgery. In certain circumstances, particularly in trauma patients, large volumes of fluid may have been consumed as alcohol and the patient may have litres of fluid within the stomach and small intestine. Patients who have a mechanical obstruction of the small intestine may also have large quantities of fluid in the small bowel. The healthy gastrointestinal tract secretes approximately 8 l of fluid per day, most of which is normally reabsorbed. However, in small-bowel obstruction very little fluid is reabsorbed and there is therefore a copious quantity of fluid present that may constitute a major threat of pulmonary aspiration following induction of anaesthesia.

Fluid may also collect in the stomach and small bowel as a result of a paralytic ileus from a variety of causes. Although the volume of fluid is usually less than in mechanical small-bowel obstruction, it still represents a copious amount and therefore a serious risk of aspiration.

Blood may also be present in the stomach as a result of either bleeding from the upper gastrointestinal tract (oesophageal varices, gastric ulceration etc.) or swallowing of blood from the nose, mouth and pharynx.

Finally, the obstetric patient with a full stomach presents a number of problems that are well described. Briefly, many obstetric procedures present as emergencies with little time for patient preparation. Endotracheal intubation may be technically more difficult than normal, and although the volumes of gastric aspirate may not be very large the consequences of aspiration of even a small amount of gastric acid and the resultant Mendehlson syndrome appear to be more severe in the obstetric patient than in others.

The specific threshold volumes and pH values of gastric contents that result in significant morbidity are not known, but a number of assumptions can be made. Morbidity may result from aspiration of the following (Kaller and Everett, 1993):

- small volumes with a very low pH, producing a chemical pneumonitis;
- large volumes of fluid of neutral pH, resulting in asphyxia, hypoxia and later infection and adult respiratory distress syndrome;
- food residues and particulate matter, resulting in airway obstruction and infection.

Clearly those patients with surgical disease resulting in large volumes of gastric fluid will be at most risk, but a number of other situations may predispose to gastric aspiration. These are shown in Table 1.

**Table 1.** Factors predisposing to gastric aspiration.

| |
|---|
| Gastric–oesophageal disease |
| Incompetent lower oesophageal sphincter (LOS) |
| Anaesthetic drugs (opioids, benzodiazepines, thiopentone, volatiles) |
| Obesity |
| Diabetes |
| Peptic ulcer disease |
| Stress |
| Pain |
| Trauma |

### *Pre-anaesthetic management*

A clinical history is essential in order to establish the nature of the problem. Information regarding recent intake of food and drink should be sought.

The nature of the meal may be relevant, because fat is cleared from the stomach more slowly than carbohydrate. It should also be remembered that gastric emptying may be slowed as a result of other factors including previous surgery (i.e. vagotomy), opioid administration and stress. In particular, the time relationship between food intake and trauma is also important. Following trauma, gastrointestinal motility may be severely impaired and trauma occurring shortly after a meal may result in food remaining in the stomach for considerably longer than 4 hours. Patients with an impaired conscious level and who are unable to give a clear history should be treated as having a full stomach.

In contrast, clear fluids are cleared relatively quickly from the stomach, and 1–2 hours may be adequate for gastric clearance of water, coffee and clear fruit juices (Maltby et al, 1986; Scarr et al, 1989).

In many situations the nature of the problem will be obvious from the surgical diagnosis, and patients with small-bowel obstruction or absent bowel sounds represent a significant risk as discussed.

### *Drainage of secretions*

Patients with mechanical intestinal obstruction and paralytic ileus should have a wide-bore nasogastric tube placed before induction of anaesthesia and gastric secretions removed by suction. This serves not only to lessen the risk of regurgitation and aspiration but also to decompress the bowel and to lessen the risk of mucosal ischaemia due to increased intraluminal pressure. Once the initial contents have been removed by suction, a drainage bag may be attached to the end of the nasogastric tube to allow free drainage.

Although large amounts of fluid may be removed, the stomach can never be emptied with certainty and therefore the patient should still be prepared for anaesthesia as if they were at risk from aspiration of gastric contents. To that end, current practice is to recommend removal of the nasogastric tube immediately before induction of anaesthesia as the presence of a nasogastric tube has been shown to reduce the effectiveness of cricothyroid pressure in preventing regurgitation of stomach contents. Frequently, the nasogastric tube will need to be repositioned after induction of anaesthesia and the airway has been secured.

### *Barrier pressure, lower oesophageal sphincter tone and intragastric pressure*

An increase in intragastric pressure (IGP) will tend to cause an increased likelihood of regurgitation. This may be opposed by the tone of the LOS. The resulting pressure is the barrier pressure (BrP), that is the pressure opposing gastric regurgitation, and is shown by the equation BrP = LOS tone − IGP (Feneck, 1998).

BrP therefore may be increased by either drugs or manoeuvres which tend to increase LOS tone and to reduce IGP. These are shown in Table 2. However, it should be noted that the net effect of suxamethonium is to

**Table 2.** Factors affecting barrier pressure.

Pharmacological

Induction agents

- Thiopentone lowers BrP. Effects of other agents unclear

Muscle relaxants

- Suxamethonium raises BrP (causes LOS tone increase by cholinergic effect, overcoming increase in IGP)
- Non-depolarizing relaxants have little effect

Anti-cholinergics

- Generally reduces BrP by relaxing LOS tone
- Atropine takes 5 min to relax LOS; no contraindication at induction

Gastrokinetics

- May increase BrP by improving gastric emptying and reducing IGP

Mechanical

Nasogastric drainage

- Increases BrP by reducing IGP if stomach very full

Posture

- Head-down tilt reduces BrP by increasing IGP but will improve drainage and avoid pulmonary contamination and soiling

Cricoid pressure

- No effect on BrP at LOS, but protects against regurgitation

increase BrP and that the onset of intravenous atropine is such that, if the drug is given at induction, LOS is not adversely affected.

### *Gastrokinetic agents*

The theoretical benefits of enhancing gastric emptying by the use of gastrokinetic agents are clear. Enhancing gastric peristalsis should enable rapid clearance of food and drink from the stomach and thereby reduce gastric contents and lessen the risk of aspiration. However, gastrokinetics may not be reliably effective in practice, and aspiration of even small volumes may cause significant pulmonary morbidity. The most commonly used drug is metoclopramide, a dopaminergie antagonist that stimulates gastric emptying, increases LOS tone, relaxes the pylorus and duodenum and has an anti-emetic effect also. An intravenous dose given 15 minutes before induction of anaesthesia will reduce the volume but not the acidity of gastric contents. Metoclopromide may be most effective in patients with large gastric fluid volumes, for example trauma, obesity, obstetrics and neurogenic delayed gastric emptying due to diabetes. However, its central dopamine antagonist effects may result in extrapyramidal side-effects. Gastrokinetic agents are absolutely contraindicated in patients with bowel obstruction.

### *Anti-emetics*

Many patients undergoing emergency surgery may require systemic analgesics, including opioids. There is a high incidence of opioid-induced nausea and vomiting, which may be as distressing as the original pain felt by the patient, and thus many patients require anti-emetics. However, the value of anti-emetic drugs in the prevention of gastric aspiration is not clear. Certainly some drugs have a combination of beneficial effects (metoclopramide), and others may reduce LOS tone and thereby reduce BrP and increase the tendency to regurgitation (e.g. anti-cholinergics). The butyrophenones (droperidol, haloperidol) are effective anti-emetics but may produce other unwanted effects including hypotension and extra-pyramidal signs.

The most effective group of anti-emetic drugs currently are the 5-hydroxytryptamine antagonists, for example odansetron and grisansetron. However, their effect on barrier pressure is not clear.

### *Antacids*

These may be particularly valuable in emergency surgery when the gastric contents are presumed to be of low volume and low pH. Oral antacids are the most effective because they increase the pH of the gastric contents immediately, and non-particulate antacids are recommended because they are thought to be less likely to cause pulmonary damage in the event of aspiration. It is possible to give 30 ml of 0.3 mol/l sodium citrate up to 15 minutes before induction, and this is effective in almost 100% of patients (Viegas et al, 1981).

The oxyntic cells secrete an isotonic solution of hydrochloric acid with a small and variable amount of sodium and potassium chloride, and secretory activity is promoted by drugs acting as agonists on the $H_2$ histamine receptors. $H_2$ receptor antagonists may therefore reduce secretory activity and cause the pH of gastric fluid to rise. This is an effective way of reducing the dangers of aspiration, provided that the $H_2$ receptor antagonists can be given long enough before anaesthesia. In practice the time lag between parenteral $H_2$ antagonist administration is rarely less than 1 hour and may be longer, although the effect may last for up to 9 hours with ranitidine (Tweedle and Nightingale, 1989). $H_2$ antagonists should not therefore be relied on to increase gastric pH before induction of anaesthesia in emergency cases because there is unlikely to be a delay of some hours before surgery. However, $H_2$ antagonists administered before induction may reduce the risks from post-extubation aspiration and therefore may still be warranted.

$H_2$ antagonists may be used in obstetric patients in prolonged labour. In this situation, the probability of an emergency instrumental delivery is increased, but the exact timing is such that it may be some hours away, thus giving $H_2$ antagonists time to be effective.

## Loss of circulating volume

Loss of circulating volume may occur as a result of the following:

- acute haemorrhage;
- loss of plasma in burned patients;
- secondary to severe dehydration in patients suffering from repetitive vomiting and failure to reabsorb gastrointestinal secretions.

### *Blood loss and replacement*

Estimating blood loss prior to emergency surgery is notoriously difficult. Reliance on simple haemodynamics may be misleading, because blood pressure may be very well maintained by peripheral vasoconstriction, and may serve to raise venous pressure also, until such time as decompensation occurs and the blood pressure falls dramatically. Induction of anaesthesia may reduce sympathetic outflow and thus vascular tone, and muscular relaxation may reduce the intra-abdominal pressure serving to maintain inferior vena caval pressure and hence right-heart filling pressures. Thus, in the hypovolaemic patient, induction of anaesthesia and muscle relaxation may be accompanied by precipitous hypotension unless adequate fluid replacement has been carried out.

Blood loss estimation in trauma patients is particularly important, because multiple trauma can add up to substantial blood losses.

Blood loss into body cavities may differ markedly in effect on general haemodynamics. Blood loss into the pericardium is poorly tolerated and may cause cardiac tamponade, classically identified by a reduction in arterial blood pressure, an increase in central venous pressure and signs of a low cardiac output such as a reduction in urine production and peripheral body temperature. Blood loss into the pleural cavity is better tolerated but will eventually cause collapse of lung tissue, an increase in intrapulmonary shunt and worsening hypoxaemia. Blood loss into the peritoneum may be prodigious before the haemodynamic effects are marked, and abdominal tenderness, or guarding and rigidity may be more apparent.

Blood loss and the resulting haemotoma formation may also be an indication for surgery, but in this setting the volume lost may be very small. Haematoma in the neck may cause airway compression and stridor, and subdural or intracranial haematoma may cause rapid and severe deterioration in concious level owing to compression and need emergency evacuation and drainage.

In the case of emergency re-operation, the amount of blood in the surgical drains may give an accurate indication of the blood volume lost, and this may be the primary indication for emergency surgery. In the case of emergency resternotomy both the pattern and the volume of chest tube drainage may be relevant.

Blood loss replacement is essential, but the scale and timing may vary. Furthermore, there is no international consensus on the question of crystalloid versus colloid replacement, but the advocates of colloid replacement therapy have now tended to include some crystalloid replacement also.

Volume replacement following blood loss has tended towards a policy of mild and limited permissive hypotension, in that this may allow surgical haemostasis to proceed more quickly and effectively. The terms ‘mild’ and ‘limited’ should be stressed; induction of anaesthesia is extremely hazardous in patients with a significantly reduced circulating volume, and if the duration of hypotension is prolonged organ failure will ensue. It is better perhaps to stress that massive volume replacement with the intention of achieving 'normal' arterial blood pressure may be counterproductive in serving to delay surgical haemostasis and increase the tendency to bleed through thrombolysis.

In the event of massive blood loss (i.e. >200 ml), packed red cells need to be given. These should be given in addition to crystalloid–colloid resuscitation, and a haematocrit of 20–25% is ideal in a young fit adult. In older patients, and those with cardiovascular disease, the ideal haematocrit should be increased to 30–35%.

Resuscitative fluids are best administered through a 5 cm wide bore (14 g) cannula sited in a peripheral vein. This will allow a flow rate of approximately 250 ml/min of crystalloid fluid at normothermia; this flow rate will be reduced by factors that increase fluid viscosity, i.e. blood, cold temperature. Intravenous fluids should be given through warming devices which serve to reduce their viscosity and hence increase their rate of delivery, and will reduce the cooling effect of the fluid on the patient. This is a particular problem in patients requiring a massive blood transfusion.

Many patients will not require blood transfusion prior to surgery, but blood and/or blood products must be available during the operation. Availability of blood varies geographically and temporally, and the distribution of blood groups within the population varies also. In the UK, 90% of the population are either blood group A or O. The time taken to process a blood sample from the patient is modest. A full blood group, antibody screen and cross-match takes 45 minutes from receipt of the blood sample, whereas a rapid group and quick-spin cross-match to exclude ABO incompatibility takes about 20 minutes. The formulation of blood offered by the laboratory varies internationally, but whole blood, SAG-M blood, plasma-reduced blood and red-cell concentrate are the most common.

### *Loss of plasma*

Loss of large quantities of plasma occurs typically in burned patients, and the amount lost may be highly significant in terms of the effect on circulating volume and haemodynamics. Plasma loss estimation and the acute management of the burned patient is highly specialized and outside the scope of this chapter. The reader is referred to the standard texts that are available. Fluid replacement therapy is vital to the pre-operative management of these patients, although in the UK there is still a debate regarding the place of crystalloid versus colloid replacement.

### *Dehydration and loss of extracellular fluid*

The stomach and small bowel secrete large volumes of fluid which is rich in hydrogen ($H^+$), sodium ($Na^+$), potassium ($K^+$) and chloride ($Cl^-$) ions. This fluid and the accompanying electrolytes are usually reabsorbed in the large bowel. However, if gastrointestinal secretions are lost either because of repetitive vomiting or as a result of iatrogenic bowel decompression and drainage via a nasogastric tube, severe dehydration, metabolic alkalosis and hypokalaemia may ensue. The dehydration may provoke circulatory collapse, and hypokalaemia may also lead to life-threatening arrhythmias. Calculation of the fluid and electrolyte losses can be made with relative ease and these can be derived from the formulae shown below (Feneck, 1998).

*Water deficit*

$$\text{body water deficit} = \text{normal body water} - \text{present body water}$$
$$\text{normal body water} = \text{body weight (kg)} \times 0.6$$
$$\text{present body water} = \frac{\text{normal serum Na} \times \text{normal body water}}{\text{present serum Na}}$$

*Sodium deficit*

$$\text{Na deficit} = (\text{normal serum Na} - \text{present serum Na}) \times \text{body weight (kg)} \times 0.2$$

*Potassium deficit*

$$\text{K losses} = (\text{normal serum K} - \text{present serum K}) \times \text{body weight (kg)} \times 0.4$$

Water and electrolyte deficiencies are often interrelated and thus considering them separately is not helpful. In all but the most complex patients, it is usual to replace lost fluid with normal saline or compound sodium lactate (Hartmann's solution), both of which have an osmolarity close to that of normal extracellular fluid (ECF) (ECF, 280–310 mOsmol/l; NaCl, 308 mOsmol/l; Hartmann's solution, 273 mOsmol/l). Water deficit can be made up by giving 5% dextrose solution (253 mOsmol/l). In most patients, extra electrolytes will be needed, particularly potassium, whatever replacement fluid is used. In diabetics, it is wise to avoid lactate-containing solutions if possible.

In addition to making up fluid deficits, fluid and electrolyte maintenance requirements must be met, but in the emergency patient both initial deficit and maintenance may need to be given simultaneously. Thus, considering a 70 kg adult,

- replacement of deficit (often 1–2 l)
- thereafter 2–4 ml/kg per hour, i.e. 140–280 ml/hour thereafter,

or

- deficit and maintenance replacement of 10–15 ml/kg per hour for the first hour (700–1000 ml) followed by 5 ml/kg per hour (350 ml/hour) thereafter.

These regimes are given only as a guideline, and obviously the losses during major bowel surgery for example will be much greater than for a simple appendicectomy.

## Pre-operative monitoring of fluids and electrolytes

The emergency patient should be appropriately monitored pre-operatively and this will be determined by both the nature of the procedure and the sickness of the patient. Whatever level of monitoring is required during the period of patient preparation, electrocardiogram, pulse oximetry and blood pressure measurements should be made in the immediate pre-induction period in all patients.

In all but the simplest of cases, volume replacement is best titrated against central venous pressure (CVP) measurements, but it is essential to remember that the CVP measurement may be artificially raised in the conscious patient owing to peripheral vasoconstriction from blood loss, pain and anxiety. Induction of anaesthesia in the peripherally vasoconstricted hypovolaemic patient may produce severe hypotension and therefore adequate circulating volume should be ensured. A CVP of 8–10 mmHg and arterial blood pressure of 60–70 mmHg mean would usually be acceptable.

The value of sophisticated haemodynamic monitoring is constantly debated. In those patients who are deemed to be seriously at risk, pre-operative pulmonary artery catheterization may be of value, particularly in patients with severe pre-existing sepsis, pulmonary hypertension or those with pulmonary oedema.

In patients requiring fluid replacement therapy, serum electrolytes should be measured, including sodium, potassium, chloride, urea, and creatinine. Abnormalities in electrolytes should be dealt with appropriately.

### *Serum sodium*

The normal value is 135–145 mmol/l. A raised serum sodium may be due to dehydration, excessive administration of sodium (usually by administration of sodium bicarbonate) or hyperaldosteronism. In the emergency setting, a serum sodium raised by dehydration is the most worrying because induction of anaesthesia in such a patient may be accompanied by severe hypotension. A low cardiac output state and vital organ hypoperfusion may already be evident.

Both the fluid depletion and the hypernatraemia may be substantially corrected by intravenous sodium-free crystalloid solution such as 5% dextrose. Usually at least 1–2 l of fluid are required.

Encouraging a diuresis will also help to correct the hypernatraemia, but excess administration of bicarbonate may be more difficult to treat, not least because the $NaHCO_3$ will have been used in the first place to treat a severe metabolic acidosis.

Hyponatraemia may occur most commonly as a result of water overload. This is often iatrogenic, caused by intravenous replacement of large volumes of fluid containing no sodium. However, it may also occur in patients with either primary (Addison disease) or secondary adrenocortical failure. Cautious replacement with twice normal NaCl may be useful. Corticosteroids will also be useful particularly in those patients suffering from steroid depletion. Severe hyponatraemia due to adrenal disease carries a very poor prognosis.

### *Serum potassium*

The normal value is 4.5–5.5 mmol/l. Serum potassium is commonly low in patients suffering from potassium losses, i.e. loss of small-bowel secretions, and in patients given clear fluids without adequate potassium supplements. Alternatively it is commonly high in patients suffering from metabolic acidosis, poor cardiovascular function and tissue perfusion or in patients given too much potassium replacement therapy or large quantities of stored blood which is rich in potassium (the potassium level in a pack of stored red cells may be as high as 7 mmol/l).

Whenever possible serum potassium should be within normal limits before induction of anaesthesia, particularly if the patient is suffering from potassium-related arrhythmias such as ventricular ectopic beats. Potassium replacement can be given by slow intravenous infusion (i.e. 20 mmol KCl diluted in at least 50 ml dextrose or normal saline and given over at least 30 minutes). However, the amount of potassium replacement required may be difficult to predict from the serum value.

In hyperkalaemia, steps may be needed to reduce serum potassium acutely before induction. These may include

- giving glucose and insulin to reduce the potassium concentration acutely,
- giving calcium salts intravenously to provide physiological antagonism for the cardiovascular effects of potassium,
- if appropriate, using a calcium–resonium enema, and
- if necessary, haemodiafiltration or haemodialysis to reduce the serum potassium.

The level of serum that is acceptable before induction of anaesthesia will be variable but may be influenced by the following:

- the presence of arrhythmias, or electrocardiographic evidence of a raised potassium level such as peaked T waves;
- the intended use of suxamethonium as a muscle relaxant, which will tend to increase serum potassium;
- in the oligo- or anuric patient further peri-operative increases in serum potassium can be expected;
- hyperventilation and the resulting hypocapnia will tend to reduce serum potassium;
- stress responses and catecholamines will tend to reduce serum potassium;
- large transfusions of stored blood will tend to increase serum potassium.

### *Serum urea and creatinine*

A high serum urea may signify dehydration, but a raised urea and creatinine constitute evidence of renal impairment. A detailed discussion of the peri-operative management of renal failure is outside the scope of this chapter, but in the emergency setting pre-renal causes are likely to be most common, and attention must be paid to optimizing the circulation. It will often be necessary to promote a diuresis by using bolus doses or infusions of diuretics including frusemide and mannitol and by optimizing both cardiac output and renal blood flow using a low-dose (2–3 μg/kg per minute) dopamine infusion, although the latter therapy is controversial. Other drugs with direct peripheral dopaminergic effects including dopexamine and fenoldopam may also have a place.

Patients with severely raised pre-operative levels of urea and creatinine will probably need mechanical renal support post-operatively even if they are still passing urine.

The necessity for frequent determinations of blood gases and electrolytes will be determined by the nature of the emergency surgery and the state of the patient. Intra-arterial catheters will allow regular blood gas and electrolyte monitoring as well as accurate blood pressure measurement and are therefore essential in the sicker patients. The pre-operative placement of central venous and peripheral arterial catheters is often valuable, but it may not be possible to delay surgery until they are placed, particularly in the patient suffering massive haemorrhage.

## PRE-EXISTING DISEASE

The presence of pre-existing disease may act as a more serious complication to the management of the emergency patient in comparison with those patients undergoing elective surgery. First, the pre-existing condition may complicate or be partly responsible for the surgical emergency, and second there is frequently little time to optimize or even to stabilize any acute deterioration in the pre-existing disease state. Nonetheless, an accurate evaluation of pre-existing disease will enable appropriate steps to be taken intra- and post-operatively, even if there is little time to optimize the patient in the pre-operative period.

### Pulmonary complications

Chronic chest disease is likely to be a major source of peri-operative morbidity, and yet there is little that can be done for the majority of emergency patients. Chest physiotherapy may be impractical owing to time constraints and the state of the patient. If there is evidence of a chest infection, broad-spectrum antibiotics should be started, but the most important aspect of emergency preparation is to drain any intrapleural blood, fluid or air by an appropriately sited chest drain. Although fluid and blood drainage may be delayed until after induction of anaesthesia, air should always be drained before induction because of the effects of intermittent positive pressure ventilation (IPPV) on the pneumothorax in the case of a bronchopleural fistula and because of the effects of nitrous oxide on the size of any air trapped in the pleural space. A bronchopleurocutaneous fistula (e.g. following trauma) may be less difficult because there is a drainage pathway for intrapleural air and a tension pneumothorax is unlikely to develop.

A post-pneumonectomy bronchopleural fistula is a relatively rare complication nowadays, but leads to drainage of fluid, frequently infected, via the pneumonectomy stump which may produce copious quantities of foul sputum and soiling of the remaining lung. The anaesthetic and surgical management is highly specialized, but pre-operation preparation would include percutaneous drainage of the pneumonectomy space, to remove as much infected fluid as possible, and antibiotics.

An acute attack of asthma may be precipitated in the emergency surgical patient, particularly those whose attacks are precipitated by psychological stress. Acute asthma should be treated whenever possible before surgery by nebulized or intravenous bronchodilators, because hypoxia will inevitably worsen during induction of anaesthesia and IPPV may produce a risk of barotrauma. However, it may be possible to treat the patient further when anaesthesia has been safely established.

In many circumstances, it may be preferable where possible to manage patients with severe chest disease undergoing emergency surgery by regional or spinal anaesthetic techniques. These techniques have little impact on the pre-operative preparation of the patient, but of course the appropriateness of the technique will have to take into account the nature of the patient and the surgery.

## Emergency surgery in patients with coexisting cardiovascular disease

Hypertension is one of the most common cardiovascular diseases, and the relationship between hypertension and morbidity in the surgical patient has been extensive studied. High levels of blood pressure may occur in emergency patients particularly if the patient is anxious and in pain.

Controlling blood pressure pre-operatively may be difficult and may in any case be achieved more easily intraoperatively. Of greater interest is the extent to which hypertension has resulted in end-organ damage, including cardiac (left ventricular hypertrophy, evidence of ischaemic heart disease) renal (raised serum creatinine) cerebrovascular (evidence of carotid disease, stroke or transient ischaemic attacks) and peripheral vascular disease. Evidence of end-organ damage as described may affect both the intraoperative and the post-operative management of the patient.

Patients with evidence of ischaemic heart disease are at greater risk from surgery than the general population, and the risks are greater for emergency surgery than for elective procedures. It would be logical to assume that the more major the surgery the greater the risk. In these patients, efforts in the peri-operative period should concentrate on aggressive cardiovascular monitoring and treatment of ischaemic episodes. The value of different types of monitoring continues to be hotly debated; there is a consensus that pulmonary artery catheters are relatively ineffective at diagnosing myocardial ischaemia, but they may be valuable in establishing the volume status of a patient with a history of cardiac disease who has lost large volumes of fluid. This may be particularly useful in preventing sudden hypotension due to vasorelaxation in a relatively hypovolaemic patient on induction.

Transoesophageal echocardiography is effective at determining left ventricular pre-load and in establishing evidence of myocardial ischaemia, but it is a more invasive monitor and a pre-operative examination will only provide a 'snapshot' of the patient's cardiac function. Electrocardiography remains the technique of choice for prolonged cardiac monitoring for myocardial ischaemia, and in patients with recent episodes of ischaemia or infarction monitoring should be continued well into the post-operative period.

The value of anti-anginal prophylaxis has become clearer recently. The use of intravenous infusions of nitrates has been extensive as anti-anginal therapy, but their value as peri-operative anti-anginal prophylaxis has not been established. However, the value of peri-operative β-adrenergic blockade has been established and it would now appear to be advisable in patients with ischaemic heart disease undergoing elective non-cardiac surgery (Mangano and the Multicenter Study of Perioperative Ischaemia Research Group, 1996). The value of β blockade in emergency patients is likely to be just as great, given the more stressful nature of the emergency situation, but effecting β blockade may be more difficult, insofar as the oral route for therapy may be unavailable, and intravenous therapy may be more difficult to achieve safely (refer also to Chapter 4 in this issue). Cardiac failure is well documented as a cause of excess morbidity and mortality in patients undergoing surgery (Goldman, 1987), and emergency surgery is likely to be of greater risk than elective surgery.

Raised jugular venous pulse, third heart sound, gallop rhythm, pulmonary crackles and radiographic evidence including cardiomegaly, pleural effusions and Kerley B lines are well understood stigmata of cardiac failure. Acute dyspnoea, inability to lie flat and radiographic evidence of pulmonary infiltrates and upper lobe-blood diversion are stigmata of acute left ventricular failure and are even more significant as indicators of a poor outcome.

In the pre-operative period, the preparation of the emergency patient should consist of supportive measures including controlled oxygen therapy and measures to reduce pulmonary venous pressure. The use of intravenous nitrates for pulmonary venodilatation may be particularly effective, but if systemic blood pressure is low nitrates alone may be poorly tolerated, and an inotropic agent (dobutamine or epinephrine) may need to be added. Alternatively, an inodilator phosphodiesterase inhibitor such as milrinone may serve to provide an increase in inotropic effect while reducing pulmonary venous pressure by venodilatation. In general, patients who are dependent on inotropioc drugs before surgery are at markedly enhanced risk in comparison with those who are effectively treated by vasodilators alone. The mildly enhanced adrenergic state associated with anaesthesia and surgery may help patients with ventricular impairment during surgery; it is in the post-operative period that cardiovascular problems commonly arise.

## Cerebral status

Little can be done to improve the cerebral status of most emergency surgery patients. However, impaired conscious level due to metabolic derangement such as diabetes (see below) or concommitant trauma (see below) should be evaluated. If there is any question of trauma or intracranial pathology, a computerized tomography or magnetic resonance imaging scan should be undertaken before surgery. The patient's neurological status should be recorded by a formal recording scale (e.g. Glasgow coma scale) both before and after surgery.

### Diabetes

Diabetic patients have an increased incidence of peripheral vascular and coronary disease as well as an increased incidence of renal disease. They are prone to infections and other problems requiring surgical intervention. Diabetics undergoing emergency surgery are therefore a high-risk group, often over 50 years of age, prone to obesity and end-organ and vascular damage complicating the delivery of safe anaesthesia. A high proportion (up to 25%) of diabetics on a surgical ward may be newly diagnosed.

The diabetogenic response to surgical stress, peripheral insulin resistance and poor diabetic control may result in severe hyperglycaemia, hyperosmolality, ketoacidosis and dehydration from osmotic diuresis even before surgery. Although complete control may not be possible before surgery, every attempt should be made to replace fluid, to control blood sugar and to replace electrolytes in the time available.

Pre-operative dehydration may be severe; up to 10 l of ECF deficit may be present. This should be corrected over the next 24 hours, preferably with half the fluid requirements being given in the first 8 hours and the remainder more slowly.

Hyperglycaemia should be corrected by intravenous insulin, which is best given by continuous intravenous infusion using a syringe pump. Fifty international units of human insulin are added to 50 ml of normal saline and infused as required, but usually between 2 and 10 units per hour, although more may be required initially. Potassium supplements will be required, and the key to safe management is to measure serum glucose and potassium levels regularly: at least half-hourly before and during emergency surgery if the patient is unstable. It is essential to achieve the best possible metabolic control before the start of surgery, because the additional surgical stress usually further disrupts diabetic control. Furthermore, severe abdominal pain in a diabetic may be caused by ketoacidosis, and the pain may disappear with effective diabetic control.

Although each diabetic must be treated and monitored individually, regimes have been described which 'clamp' 90% of diabetics at between 6 and 12 mmol/l of glucose (Alberti and Thomas, 1979), for example the following:

- 50 U insulin in a 50 ml syringe, run at 2 U/hour (Humulin S);
- 100 ml/hour of 5% dextrose;
- if blood glucose concentration is less than 6 mmol/l, increase rate of fluid administration to 200 ml/hour;
- if blood glucose concentration is more than 12 mmol/l, increase insulin by 1 U/hour.

Potassium chloride is added to the dextrose fluid as required.

## Renal failure

Renal failure patients requiring emergency surgery will usually demonstrate coexisting uraemia, anaemia, hyperkalaemia and metabolic acidosis. Either hyper- or hypovolaemia may be present, depending on whether the surgical emergency entails fluid losses and whether the patient has been recently dialysed. Hypovolaemia should be corrected with normal saline; there will frequently be no time to remove excess fluid by dialysis, but cardiovascular instability is less likely in the hypervolaemic patient during induction of anaesthesia. However, serum potassium may be elevated, and if suxamethonium is used the potassium level may increase further, giving rise to arrhythmias. The serum potassium should be lowered if possible (e.g. by intravenous glucose and insulin), consideration given to using a non-depolarizing relaxant for intubation if possible and calcium chloride should be available for intravenous administration.

Patients with chronic renal failure may demonstrate a coagulopathy due to disorders of platelet function and long-standing severe anaemia. Neither of these should be aggressively treated in the pre-operative period unless absolutely essential. The disorder of platelet function usually improves with dialysis, and anaemia in chronic renal failure is usually well tolerated owing to the increased cardiac output and elevated red cell concentrations of 2,3-diphosphoglycerate. Blood transfusion may serve to cause further bone marrow depression, but when acute blood loss has occurred transfusion should not be withheld.

## The jaundiced patient

Although these patients may present for virtually any surgical procedure, anaesthesia is more commonly required for surgery on the hepatobiliary system. Pre-operative assessment of the emergency patient needs to take into account the following:

- the presence and grading of hepatic coma;
- the presence of ascites;
- the serum bilirubin;
- the serum albumin;
- the prothrombin time.

The main factors to assess in the pre-operative period are as follows:

- the need for fresh frozen plasma and vitamin K, depending on the prothrombin time;
- measures to counteract the peri-operative development of acute renal failure (this is a well-documented entity in jaundiced patients, and suggested aetiological factors include hypoxia, decrease in renal blood flow, toxic effects of bilirubin on the kidney and the effect of intestinal endotoxins).

A urinary catheter should be passed and, if the pre-operative serum bilirubin is between 20 and 140 μmol/l, a urinary output of 50 ml/hour should be maintained. Mannitol (10%) is best for this purpose, given as a bolus of 100–500 ml according to the CVP and maintained as an infusion during and after surgery. Although other drugs have been used (frusemide, dopamine), mannitol appears to be more effective.

### The burst abdomen

Wound breakdown may be primarily associated with infection, although surgical and anaesthetic technique and the general health of the patient may be influential.

Resuturing of abdominal wounds, the so-called 'burst abdomen', is important in that they are notoriously difficult to assess and although they may be listed as minor cases they often involve bowel stasis, a 'full stomach' and fluid and electrolyte disturbance. If a small piece of prolapsed omentum or bowel is visible, a full resuturing is likely and the patient should be worked up as for a formal laparotomy.

### Acute vascular emergency

The emergency resection of any arterial aneurysm is likely to be a prolonged operation requiring extensive blood transfusion, fluid and electrolyte replacement, possible cardiovascular support and a period of post-operative intensive or high-dependency care. Emergency embolectomy is more subtle. The patient frequently presents with a cold pulseless limb, and there is often time to ensure that the patient is partially prepared before surgery. In addition to acute surgical parameters, time should be spent trying to identify the source of the embolism (new atrial fibrillation, left ventricular thrombus, valvular vegetations etc.) because this will give insights into the patient's medical status and also help to direct treatment and monitoring in the post-operative period.

Acute mesenteric embolus presents as an abdominal emergency, often after myocardial infarction or cardiac surgery. The condition develops as an acute abdomen and, after a number of hours, it becomes clear that a laparotomy is inevitable. At this stage, embolectomy or bowel resection is rarely curative and results are poor. What is needed is a more effective way of establishing the diagnosis earlier, but so far results have not been encouraging.

### Trauma

There is a considerable literature on the management of the traumatized patient which cannot be covered in this text. Emergency trauma care can be regarded as a control system (Oakley and Baskett, 1996). The patient has sustained damage to anatomical structures with the consequence of disturbance to physiological systems. The principles of trauma management can be generalized as anatomical structure control and physiological system control.

Although the main priority is the acute clinical management of the trauma situation, this should include an assessment of the cause. Falls, loss of consciousness while driving etc. may be caused by arrhythmias, acute myocardial infarction, stroke or transient ischaemic attack, convulsions and other factors, all of which will be relevant to the peri-operative management of the patient.

Many of the features of pre-operative trauma management have been described under general headings. Management of the full stomach and blood and fluid loss will apply to all trauma patients. Detailed examination of the chest is necessary, and where appropriate chest drains should be sited to drain blood and air from the pleural space. An initial Glasgow coma score should be recorded, and repeated if necessary. In head trauma, the following should be sought specifically:

- evidence of base of skull fracture, including cerebrospinal fluid rhinorrhea, peri-orbital haematomata, bleeding from the external auditory meatus, bruising over the mastoid process;
- evidence of mandibular fracture (masseter spasm, sublingual haematoma);
- evidence of maxillary fracture and backwards displacement.

Adequate oxygenation, pain control, fluid and electrolyte replacement and haemodynamic stabilization are central to the successful pre-operative management of trauma patients.

## REFERENCES


Adams AP, Hewitt PB & Grande CM (1998) General principles of emergency anaesthesia. In Adams AP, Hewitt PB & Grande CM (eds) *Emergency Anaesthesia*, 2nd edn, pp 1–11. London: Arnold.

Alberti KG & Thomas DJ (1979) The management of diabetes during surgery. *British Journal of Anaesthesia* **51:** 693–710.

Feneck RO (1998) Abdominal surgery. In Adams AP, Hewitt PB & Grande CM (eds) *Emergency Anaesthesia*, 2nd edn, pp 121–139. London: Arnold.

Goldman L (1987) Multifactorial index of cardiac risk in non-cardiac surgical procedures: 10 year status report. *Journal of Cardiothoracic and Vascular Anesthesia* **1:** 237–242.

Kaller SK & Everett LL (1993) Potential risks and preventive measures for pulmonary aspiration; new concepts in preoperative guidelines. *Anesthesia and Analgesia* **77:** 171–182.

Mangano DT and the Multicenter Study of Perioperative Ischaemia Research Group (1996) Effect of atenolol on mortality and cardiovascular morbidity after non-cardiac surgery. *New England Journal of Medicine* **335(23):** 1713–1720.

Maltby JR, Sutherland AD, Sale JP et al (1986) Preoperative oral fluids; is a five hour fast justified prior to elective surgery? *Anesthesia and Analgesia* **65:** 1112–1116.

Oakley PA & Baskett PJF (1996) General management of the traumatized patient. In Prys-Roberts C & Brown BR (eds) *International Practice of Anaesthesia*, vol. 2, chap. 124, pp 1–24. Oxford: Butterworth–Heinemann.

Scarr M, Maltby JR, Jani K et al (1989) Volume and acidity of residual gastric fluid after oral fluid ingestion before elective ambulatory surgery. *Canadian Medical Association Journal* **141:** 1151–1154.

Tweedle D & Nightingale P (1989) Anaesthesia and gastrointestinal surgery. *Acta Chirurgica Scandinavica* **55 (supplement):** 131–139.

Viegas OJ, Ravindian RS & Shumacker CA (1981) Gastric fluid pH in patients receiving sodium citrate. *Anesthesia and Analgesia* **60:** 521–523.

9

# Pre-operative anaemia and polycythaemia

HANS GOMBOTZ MD

Associate Professor

*Department of Anaesthesiology and Intensive Care Medicine, University of Graz, Auenbruggerplatz 29, A-8036 Graz, Austria*

Alterations in haemoglobin are associated with increased risk of cardiovascular events not only in normal life but especially in the peri-operative setting. Anaemia as well as polycythaemia are symptoms of an underlying pathology and need further diagnostic evaluation for adequate treatment. Specific treatment of pre-operative anaemia is indicated, because simple transfusion of allogeneic blood does not necessarily reduce post-operative morbidity and mortality. Also, in patients with polycythaemia a reduction of elevated haemoglobin levels is essential to avoid complications due to hyperviscosity. In all patients the risk of allogeneic transfusion of blood products has to be calculated and alternative strategies should be taken into consideration. However, those methods have to be performed in a comprehensive multimodality programme adapted to the actual transfusion requirements, the patients' individual needs, the equipment available and the experience of the responsible physicians.

**Key words:** anaemia; polycythaemia; allogeneic transfusion; autologous transfusion; erythropoietin; blood conservation.

In the peri-operative setting intra- and post-operative changes in haemoglobin may become enormous compared with normal life and may make heavy demands on the compensatory mechanisms of the body. Although the isolated pre-operative risk of haemoglobin abnormalities is difficult to determine and to separate from the risk of surgery as well as the underlying pathology, it has to be weighed against the risk of delaying surgery for adequate treatment if feasible.

## PRE-OPERATIVE ANAEMIA

Anaemia is one of the most common symptoms in clinical medicine and is frequently the key to an unknown and unsuspected primary diagnosis. Patients with low haemoglobin should probably undergo further investigations before elective surgery and adequate treatment are considered.

*Baillière's Clinical Anaesthesiology*—
Vol. 12, No. 3, September 1998
ISBN 0–7020–2536–4
0950–3501/98/030451 + 19 $12.00/00

Criteria for anaemia as defined by the World Health Organisation are haemoglobin values <13 g/dl in men and <12 g/dl in women for persons older than 14 years living at sea level (Anonymous, 1968). In the general population of the western hemisphere there is an estimated increase of 10–18 cases with anaemia per 1000 patients identified by primary care physicians (McPhee, 1982). Anaemia is rare in children, but the incidence of anaemia rises with age and is higher in men than in women whereby even mild degrees of anaemia are associated with reduced survival (Ania et al, 1997). During the lifetime the average haemoglobin is higher in men than in women with a sharp decrease over the age of 70 years. In contrast, in women there is a constant increase of haemoglobin after 50 years of age followed by a slight decrease over 70 years (Figure 1) (Gagnon et al, 1994).

In the elderly population acute blood loss due to surgery was found to be the leading cause of anaemia (Ania et al, 1997). The survival rate among patients in whom anaemia followed surgery was better than in non-surgical cases, a finding which may point out the importance of the underlying pathology but also the importance of anaemia as an indicator of any serious disease. Systematic pre-operative screening of older people for haemoglobin abnormalities, therefore, may serve as a useful and cost-effective tool, but it has also to be shown that adequate treatment may have a favourable effect on quality of life and survival.

Common aetiologies of anaemia are iron deficit, physiological anaemia of pregnancy, sickle cell anaemia, pernicious anaemia, anaemia of chronic disease, haemolytic anaemia, surgical blood loss or even anaemia due to frequent phlebotomies because of autologous pre-donation. Sudden blood loss due to trauma or surgery or other losses usually in the gastrointestinal tract cause acute anaemia. The most common cause of chronic anaemia is iron deficiency followed by anaemia of chronic disease. Anaemia of chronic disease occurs in the presence of chronic or acute infections or inflammatory disease or in association with renal failure or liver disease. In a cohort of 2183 orthopaedic patients 19.8% of the female patients and 12%

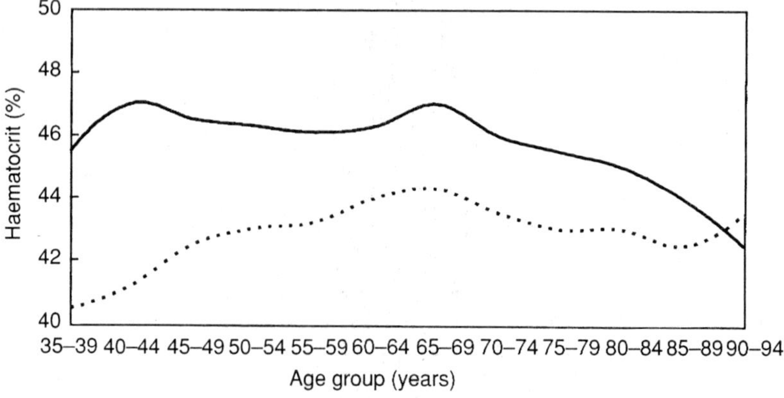


**Figure 1.** Haemoglobin changes over life-time in men (——) and women (•••••) (Gagnon et al, 1994).

of the male patients had a baseline haematocrit of less than 34% (Mercuriali and Inghilleri, in press). In patients with rheumatoid arthritis the percentage of patients with low baseline haematocrit increased to 25% and in patients suffering from cancer to 30%. Those patients were unable to donate a sufficient amount of autologous blood and were at risk of allogeneic transfusion. Furthermore, almost 40% of elderly patients with primary hip fracture had pre-operative haemoglobin values of less than 12 g/dl (Carson et al, 1998). In contrast to elderly people, pre-operative anaemia is rare in children but is more likely to occur in those less than 1 year of age (Hackmann et al, 1991).

Iron deficiency causes microcytic hypochromic anaemia with low ferritin levels (<12 μg/l), a decrease in transferrin saturation (<16%) and a rise in free erythrocyte porphyrins or zinc protoporphyrin, which can readily be measured by fluorometry. Zinc protoporphyrin is recommended as a feasible and inexpensive pre-donation test to determine a subset of donors with iron deficit (Harthoorn et al, 1998). However, fluorometric zinc protoporphyrin determination was only of limited value in a cohort of patients undergoing pre-donation of autologous blood (Posch et al, 1994).

Anaemia of chronic disease is characterized as a mild-to-moderate normocytic anaemia with low transferrin saturation, high transferrin concentration and high serum ferritin levels (Means and Krantz, 1992). Normal serum transferrin receptor concentration may be used to distinguish these patients from patients with iron deficit (Ferguson et al, 1992). The pathophysiology of cancer-related anaemia is not fully understood and is probably due to different causes (Spivak, 1994). It is characterized by excessive release of inflammatory cytokines and variable degrees of erythropoietin production and worsened by blood loss and by depressive effects of chemotherapy or radiation. This type of anaemia develops slowly and initially unnoticed and is usually mild to moderate with haemoglobin values between 8 and 10 g/dl. Extensive cancer anaemia, however, is indicative of poor prognosis. Patients with anaemia due to rheumatoid arthritis have lower erythropoietin levels than those with simple iron deficit but also frequently have coexistent iron deficit (Pincus et al, 1990; Vreugdenhil et al, 1992). Anaemia due to rheumatoid arthritis is usually mild and well tolerated but anaemia indicates a more serious course of the disease which is augmented by complications of concomitant drug therapy. When surgery has to be performed anaemia of chronic disease may worsen dramatically. Blood conservation methods may become impossible or ineffective and allogeneic transfusion cannot be avoided. The relative erythropoietin deficiency found in patients with rheumatoid arthritis and cancer as well as human immunodeficiency virus (HIV) with zidovudine therapy has led to the successful use of recombinant erythropoietin in these patients (Pincus et al, 1990; Abels, 1992). In patients with chronic renal failure anaemia is caused by an absolute or relative deficiency, but many additional factors such as iron deficit, decreased survival of red cells or gastrointestinal bleeding may worsen anaemia. Treatment of the anaemia of progressive renal failure with recombinant human erythropoietin has become the standard of care in recent years (Eschbach et al, 1989).

## Risk of peri-operative anaemia

The pathophysiological consequences of anaemia are a reduction in the oxygen-carrying capacity leading to profound physiological adjustment, primarily of the cardiovascular system (Messmer, 1981; Spahn et al, 1994). According to Poiseuille's law the reduction of viscosity due to the reduction of haemoglobin causes a significant decrease in peripheral vascular resistance. This phenomenon is more prominent at the low shear rates in the microcirculatory system. As a consequence, improved microcirculation augments venous return, causing an increase in cardiac output mainly by augmenting stroke volume (Messmer et al, 1986; van Iterson et al, 1995). The increase of cardiac output gradually increases with the degree of haemodilution and initially causes an increase (down to a haemoglobin level of 28%) followed by a decrease of the oxygen transport capacity. Peripheral vasodilatation plays a minor role, and the autonomic nervous system is not affected in humans (Spahn et al, 1996a). As under normal conditions oxygen extraction of the myocardium is almost complete, myocardial perfusion has to increase sufficiently to compensate for a decrease in arterial oxygen content. This augmentation of the coronary blood flow is out of proportion to the increase in cardiac output and is secondary to coronary vasodilatation (Jan and Chien, 1977). This reduction in coronary reserve becomes more important in the presence of tachycardia, decreased mean arterial pressure, critical aortic stenosis or left ventricular hypertrophy (Crystal et al, 1988). Therefore, the minimum safe haemoglobin level may also be defined as the haemoglobin level at which coronary blood flow can no longer increase sufficiently to meet the myocardial oxygen demand. There is also a significant increase in cerebral blood flow in normocapnia but blood flow to other organs increases only modestly or not at all.

Decreasing oxygen delivery with constant oxygen consumption leads to an increase in arteriovenous $O_2$ difference by increasing $O_2$ extraction. The increased peripheral oxygen extraction indeed plays an important adaptive role when haemoglobin drops below 25% (Von Restorff et al, 1975). The inability to exercise this compensatory mechanism in different vascular beds may limit the application of normovolaemic haemodilution (NHD), for example in patients with arteriosclerotic disease. The rightward shift of the oxyhaemoglobin curve caused by an increase of 2,3-diphosphoglycerate (2,3-DPG) facilitates the release of $O_2$ from the haemoglobin to tissue at any given blood $O_2$ tension. Although an increase of 2,3-DPG 90 min after the start of NHD in animal studies was shown, this mechanism is probably more important for chronic anaemia (Sunder-Plassmann et al, 1975).

The risk of anaemia adds to the risk of surgery and the risk of the underlying disease, whereby the specific cause of anaemia may have further influence on outcome. A patient with anaemia secondary to neoplasm and concomitant malnutrition is at much greater risk than an otherwise healthy patient with normovolaemia secondary to blood loss. Normovolaemia is a precondition for the tolerance of anaemia and there is no doubt that peri-operatively induced normovolaemic anaemia is better tolerated than chronic anaemia due to an underlying disease. The tolerance to intra- and post-operative anaemia is dependent on type and duration of anaemia, the baseline haemoglobin (better red cell mass), the patient's cardiovascular status and the perisurgical blood loss.

In a retrospective cohort study Carson et al (1996) investigated the natural history and the consequences of peri-operative anaemia uninfluenced by transfusion in 1958 patients undergoing non-cardiac surgery. They found an increased risk of morbidity and mortality in patients with low pre-operative haemoglobin levels, which was more pronounced in patients with concomitant cardiovascular disease, i.e. history of angina pectoris, congestive heart failure, myocardial infarction or history of peripheral vascular disease (Figure 2). A peri-operative decline in haemoglobin of 2 g/dl or less was not associated with an increased risk of death; the risk of death was highest in patients with cardiovascular disease combined with a decline of haemoglobin of 4 g/dl. Although moderate haemodilutional anaemia could be safely produced in elderly patients and in patients with coronary artery disease, low intraoperative haemoglobin values were shown to increase the risk of mortality even in situations where the patients' tolerance to anaemia may be strongly improved, for example during cardiopulmonary bypass (Spahn et al, 1996a,b; Fang et al, 1997). In this situation the heart is relieved of its burden to compensate for anaemia and cardiac output is controlled by the heart–lung machine. Hypotensive anaesthesia combined with anaemia may involve risks not warranted by the possible benefits of blood conservation as a result of major decreases in calculated oxygen delivery to critical tissue beds such as renal cortex and retina (Plewes and Farhi, 1985; Dong et al, 1986). In patients after infra-inguinal vascular surgery a haemoglobin level of <28% was significantly associated with myocardial ischaemia and morbid cardiac events, and after cardiac surgery anaemia beyond the second post-operative day could also be identified as a predictor of mortality in elderly patients (Nelson et al, 1993; Rady et al, 1998).

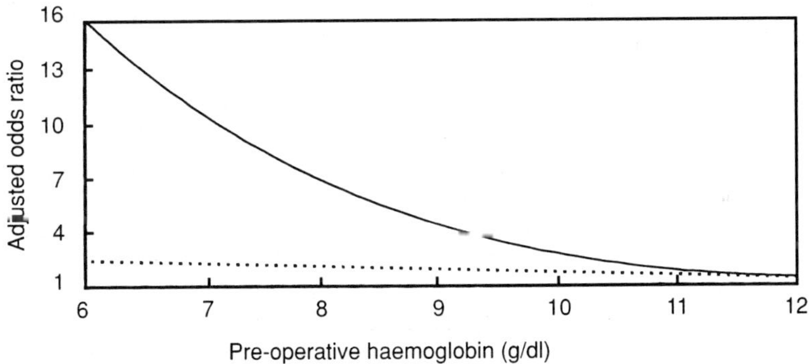


**Figure 2.** Morbidity and mortality in surgical patients with (——) and without (•••••) cardiovascular disease refusing blood transfusions. Reproduced from Carson et al (1996) Effect of anaemia and cardiovascular disease on surgical mortality and morbidity. *Lancet* **348:** 1055–1060, with permission from The Lancet Ltd.

## Probability of receiving allogeneic transfusions

The need for transfusion of red cells is the result of the difference between peri-operative and tolerable blood loss. Peri-surgical blood loss is dependent on the type of surgical procedure, accuracy of surgical technique and coagulation status as well as the applicability of specific blood-saving measures. The amount of blood loss which can be tolerated by the individual patient is mainly a function of the cardiopulmonary status and the pre-operative total circulatory red cell mass. In other words, pre-operative anaemia is a strong predictor of the need for red cell transfusions (Faris et al, 1996; Nuttall et al, 1996; Larocque et al, 1997).

Substantial surgical blood loss (e.g. more than 500 ml in adult patients) increases the risk of morbidity and mortality whereby the adverse effect of blood loss is larger in patients with low pre-operative haemoglobin levels (Table 1) (Carson et al, 1988). In a retrospective survey in Jehovah's Witness patients Viele and Weiskopf (1994) suggested that survival without transfusion is possible at low haemoglobin concentrations, while mortality with an unknown incidence is encountered at haemoglobin concentrations below 5 g/dl. With an estimated surgical blood loss of less than 500 ml combined with pre-operative haemoglobin levels of greater than 8 g/dl no mortality was found in another retrospective survey in Jehovah's Witness patients (Spence et al, 1990).

The main problem of haemoglobin-based recommendations is their lack of generalizability. Haemoglobin as a single parameter cannot be recommended, either as need for treatment of anaemia or as a decision to transfuse in elective surgery. Some patients can tolerate very low haemoglobin levels (Weiskopf et al, 1998) while others will require supranormal values to survive (Nelson et al, 1993), but there is no justification for the traditional 10 g/dl of haemoglobin or 30% of haematocrit rule anymore. Furthermore, the tolerable haemoglobin level should automatically be considered an acceptable level for all patients. Decisions about the acceptable pre-operative haemoglobin should take into account the cardiovascular and pulmonary status and the operative blood loss as well as the patient's initial red cell mass, with respect to which special symptoms of anaemia have to be considered.

**Table 1.** Risk of morbidity and mortality (odds ratio) due to baseline haemoglobin and peri-operative blood loss shown as decline in haemoglobin in patients with and without cardiovascular disease. Reproduced from Carson et al (1996) Effect of anaemia and cardiovascular disease on surgical mortality and morbidity. *Lancet* **348:** 1055–1060, with permission from The Lancet Ltd.

| Pre-operative haemoglobin(g/dl) | Decline of 2.0–3.9 g/dl | |
|---|---|---|
| | No cardiovascular disease | Cardiovascular disease |
| 6.0–6.9 | 24.1 (3.1–195.8) | 216.1 (19.3–240.4) |
| 7.0–7.9 | 14.2 (2.6–81.2) | 88.2 (11.8–656.4) |
| 8.0–8.9 | 8.30 (2.1–33.7) | 36.0 (7.2–179.3) |
| 9.0–9.9 | 4.90 (1.8–14.0) | 14.7 (4.4–49.0) |
| 10.0–10.9 | 2.89 (1.5–5.8) | 6.0 (2.7–13.4) |
| 11.0–11.9 | 1.70 (1.2–2.4) | 2.5 (1.6–3.7) |
| ⩾12.0 | Reference | Reference |

For elective surgery the maximum blood order schedule (MSBOS) given by the hospital's transfusion committee may be taken into consideration to identify operations with low transfusion requirements (Friedman et al, 1976). Patients with elective surgery only requiring type and screening procedures are not candidates for transfusion and should be discouraged from pre-depositing autologous blood. However, the MSBOS does not consider post-operative transfusions or the baseline red cell mass and cardiovascular condition of the individual patient. A more reliable approach in determining transfusion requirements may be a retrospective or better a prospective search for transfusion requirements (Audet et al, 1996). On the basis of their database, Laroque et al (1997) calculated a simple point score system to predict the likelihood of transfusion to optimize further autologous blood donation in high-risk patients. Mercuriali's algorithm, which is based on the schedule of optimal pre-operative collection of autologous blood (Axelrod et al, 1989; Mercuriali and Intaglietta, 1996), takes into account predicted blood loss determined through a constantly updated retrospective analysis of the real blood loss per surgical operation occurring in patients operated on in the previous 6–12 months minus the blood loss the patient can tolerate. On the basis of those calculations, the best transfusion strategy for the individual patient can be selected (Table 2).

**Table 2.** Calculations to estimate intra- and post-operative transfusion requirements.

| |
|---|
| Estimated RBC loss = PBV × ($Hct_{preop}$ − $Hct_{POD5}$) + RBC transfused (ml) |
| Tolerated RBC loss = (PBV × $Hct_{preop}$) − (PBV × $Hct_{min,\ accepted}$) |
| Transfusion needs = estimated blood loss − tolerated blood loss |
| where Hct is the haematocrit, RBC is the red blood cell volume and PBV is the predicted blood volume |

Modified from Mercuriali and Intaglietta (1996, *Current Medical Research Opinion* **13:** 465–478).

## Treatment of pre-operative anaemia

There is a lot of controversy and uncertainty about the adequate treatment of peri-operative anaemia which is also reflected in a number of reports about inappropriate transfusion practice even at leading academic institutions (Hebert et al, 1998; Stover et al, 1998). Although national transfusion guidelines are available in many countries, controlled studies have not been performed to determine the haemoglobin concentration at which red blood cell transfusion improves clinical outcome. In previous studies physiological variables such as oxygen transport capacity and metabolic response instead of clinical endpoints such as morbidity and mortality were examined. Not surprisingly, only few relevant data about the impact of red cell transfusions on outcome are available and most of them have been done with intensive care unit patients. In a recent study in 4470 critically ill patients, patients with lower haemoglobin values and with frequent transfusions died. In patients with cardiac disease a trend to lower mortality rates was found when given 1–3 or 4–6 units of allogeneic red cells, a finding which could not be confirmed in the surgical population (Hebert et al, 1997).

At least in patients with haemoglobin levels of 8 g/dl or higher the simple transfusion of red cells does not appear to lower the risk of 30 or 90 day morbidity and mortality but exposes the patients to the risk of allogeneic blood transfusions per se (Table 3) (Carson et al, 1998). Furthermore, at least in acute situations, because of acquired storage lesions red cell transfusion might impede or even worsen regional oxygen supply (Marik and Sibbald, 1993; Fitzgerald et al, 1997). Apart from patients with bleeding complications, who normally have to be operated on as soon as possible, patients with iron deficit and patients with anaemia of chronic disease especially those with cancer or rheumatoid arthritis are of special interest. If the cause of anaemia is clearly identified and if the clinical condition of the patient permits sufficient time for these agents to promote erythropoiesis, specific treatment with medications such as iron, vitamin $B_{12}$, folic acid or erythropoietin is recommended instead of blood transfusions.

**Table 3.** Effect of allogeneic transfusion on morbidity and mortality in elderly patients with primary hip fracture. Reproduced from Carson et al (1998) Perioperative blood transfusion and postoperative mortality. *Journal of the American Medical Association* **279:** 199–205.

| Trigger (haemoglobin g/dl) | Transfused | | Non-transfused | |
|---|---|---|---|---|
| | *N* | Mortality *N* (%) | *N* | Mortality *N* (%) |
| <7.0 | 204 | 16 (7.8) | 10 | 3 (30) |
| 7.0–7.9 | 810 | 44 (5.4) | 96 | 5 (5.2) |
| ***8.0–8.9*** | ***1620*** | ***78 (4.8)*** | ***623*** | ***22 (3.5)*** |
| ***9.0–9.9*** | ***854*** | ***49 (5.8)*** | ***1355*** | ***61 (4.5)*** |
| 10.0–10.9 | 144 | 9 (6.3) | 1429 | 59 (4.1) |
| 11.0–11.9 | 47 | 1 (2.1) | 941 | 40 (4.3) |
| ⩾12 | 20 | 0 (0.0) | 634 | 15 (2.4) |
| Total | 3699 | 197 (5.3) | 5088 | 205 (4.0) |

In patients with chronic renal disease the use of erythropoietin is well established and has led not only to a dramatic decrease of allogeneic transfusion requirements but also to a significant improvement of quality of life in this particular group of patients (Eschbach et al, 1989). The recognition of an iron deficiency is of special importance when erythropoietin therapy can be expected (Mercuriali et al, 1997). The response to treatment with erythropoietin in the presence of iron deficit is inversely correlated with the degree of anaemia but not impaired. Unresponsive patients may become responsive after correction of functional iron deficit. A special problem in those patients, which often makes iron supplementation necessary, is the possibility of a functional iron deficit, i.e. normal iron stores but inadequate iron supply to the bone marrow (Drueke et al, 1997). Nowadays renal patients are well controlled, undergo surgery with acceptable pre-operative haemoglobin levels and normally do not need additional treatment apart from their treatment with erythropoietin throughout the peri-operative period.

Outside the setting of renal disease erythropoietin is indicated in patients with defective endogeneous erythropoietin production, which includes patients with anaemia of chronic disease due to cancer or rheumatoid arthritis but also HIV patients and patients undergoing chemotherapy or patients after organ transplantation receiving cyclosporin. As for renal anaemia, recombinant human erythropoietin is approved for the treatment of anaemia in several categories of patients in many countries. After exclusion of other correctable causes of anaemia, erythropoietin treatment has to be adapted to the underlying disease and the responsiveness of the patient (Cazzola et al, 1997). Patients with a haemoglobin level of less than 10 g/dl and erythropoietin levels of less than 100 mU/ml may have a blunted erythropoietin production and be responsive to erythropoietin therapy. In patients with rheumatoid arthritis subcutaneous erythropoietin supplemented by intravenous iron has been shown to be as effective and well tolerated as higher doses of erythropoietin administered intravenously and also supplemented by intravenous iron (Mercuriali et al, 1997). Although there is a striking enhancement of iron absorption following regular erythropoietin administration in normal subjects, which is related to the combined effect of diminished iron stores and augmented erythropoiesis (Skikne and Cook, 1992), erythropoietin treatment produces a 'functional' iron deficit, and despite concomitant intravenous administration of iron saccharate there is still a decrease of plasma ferritin levels (Kulier et al, 1993). In patients with inadequate or insufficient iron stores, the response to erythropoietin is blunted, or higher dosages of the drug are necessary (Mercuriali et al, 1997). Therefore, adequate monitoring of iron metabolism is important but in clinical routine often difficult to achieve (Vreugdenhil et al, 1990). Additional measurement of reticulocyte maturity fraction with flow cytometry may become helpful for identifying iron deficiency and optimization of erythropoietin treatment (Sowade et al, 1997a).

## PRE-OPERATIVE BLOOD CONSERVATION PLANNING

On the basis of precise surgical technique and reduction of diagnostic and interventional blood loss as well as strict transfusion regimens, pre-operative deposition of autologous blood and pre-operative treatment with recombinant human erythropoietin have become cornerstones in the concepts for reducing allogeneic transfusion requirements. Blood conservation methods have to be applied according to the experience of the responsible physicians and the equipment available and to be checked subsequently with regard to their efficacy and cost effectiveness. Only a comprehensive multimodality blood conservation programme can significantly decrease bleeding and need for allogeneic transfusion in a safe and cost-effective manner (Gombotz and Kulier, 1995; Helm et al, 1998).

### Pre-deposition of autologous blood

In recent years pre-deposition of autologous blood has become standard in certain procedures with a surgical blood loss of more than 1000 ml and has led to a dramatic decrease of homologous transfusion requirements. Pre-deposition of autologous blood is still underutilized because the logistics is not simple and may be complicated by a number of factors. It is difficult to organize, and there is a high psychological and physiological demand for the patient (Figure 3). Moreover, pre-deposition of autologous blood is expensive, because it has to be processed and tested in the same way as homologous blood. The units tested seropositive have to be discharged and the patients concerned to be excluded from further donations in accordance with the rules of the official health authorities in many countries. As the need for blood transfusion is not always predictable in the individual patient, a number of autologous units have to be wasted. Those units cannot be 'carried over' for homologous use. On the other hand, 10–30% of all autologous donors still receive homologous blood, for which anaemia (haematocrit <39%) is the most important predictor (Figure 4) (Nuttall et al, 1996; Goodnough et al, 1997; Mercuriali and Inghilleri, in press).

Because of the frequent phlebotomies during pre-donation a number of patients may not only become anaemic and consequently be unable to donate the amount of blood initially planned but also have a markedly increased incidence of allogeneic transfusion with its associated risks (Kanter et al, 1996). In autologous blood donors with a normal iron status, the use of supplemental oral iron does not affect erythropoiesis and is insufficient in maintaining iron stores (Biesma et al, 1992). Furthermore, autologous blood donation is not as cost effective as most accepted medical practices. Its cost effectiveness can be substantially improved by the avoidance of overcollection and overtransfusion of autologous blood (Etchason et al, 1995; Mercuriali and Intaglietta, 1996; Chun et al, 1997; Goh et al, 1997; Larocque et al, 1997). Pre-donation is well tolerated and side-effects

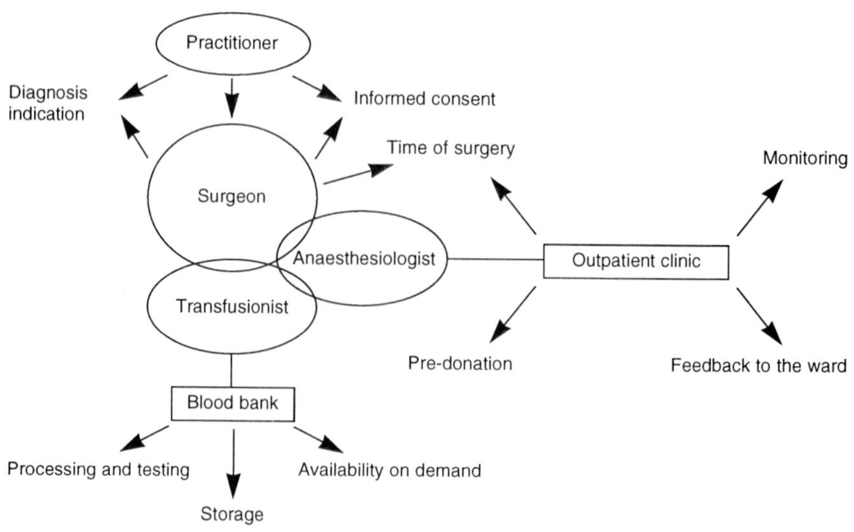


**Figure 3.** Organizing pre-deposition of autologous blood.

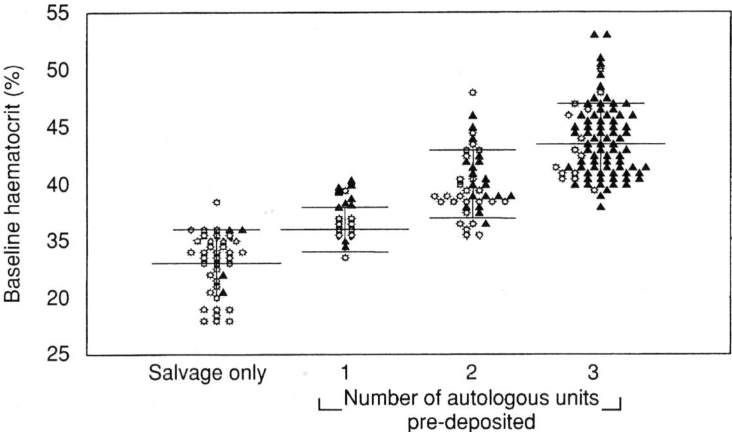


**Figure 4.** Relationship of baseline haemoglobin to the number of autologous units collected and the ability to cover transfusion needs exclusively with the use of autologous blood (Mercuriali and Inghilleri, in press): ✿, patients transfused with autologous and allogeneic blood; ▲, patients transfused with autologous blood only.

are rare and comparable with those of allogeneic donors even in high-risk autologous donors (McVay et al, 1990; Hillyer et al, 1994). Very severe complications leading to hospital stay are infrequent in all types of blood donation, but nearly 12 times as likely in autologous blood donors. Their occurrence may be associated with significant morbidity and cost (Popovsky et al, 1995). In patients with coronary artery disease there is a risk of worsening myocardial ischaemia (Nelson et al, 1993), but no demonstrable effect could be shown using Holter monitoring devices (van Dyck et al, 1994; Kasper et al, 1997a). In cardiac patients simultaneous replacement of the volume donated with colloids or crystalloids may weaken the drop in blood pressure and increase in heart rate especially after donation (Spiess et al, 1992). Logistic errors are not infrequent in autologous donation programs. In a Canadian survey the most frequent errors were made in labelling and component preparation. Errors were more frequent if components were produced when units were drawn in hospitals for interhospital transfer or when units were shipped between Red Cross centres (Goldman et al, 1997).

The basic mechanism of pre-deposition of autologous blood is the stimulation of the endogeneous erythropoiesis to increase the total amount of autologous red cells. In fact, there is an increase of endogenous erythropoietin levels, but the endogenous transfusion trigger (the haemoglobin level below which the plasma erythropoietin unequivocally increases) is below 10.5 g/dl, a level which is rarely reached during pre-deposition of autologous blood. A net gain of red cells of about 200 ml within 2 weeks can be expected and amounts to about 2/3 of the volume donated (Mercuriali and Intaglietta, 1996; Kasper et al, 1997b). A simple strategy to augment red cell volume by pre-donation is to donate as long before surgery as possible and at short intervals (Lorentz et al, 1992; Toy et al, 1994). In contrast, autologous donations 2 weeks before surgery were associated with a higher incidence of allogeneic transfusions (Larsen et al, 1994). Additional stimulation with recombinant erythropoietin in non-anaemic patients is effective in preventing the decrease of haemoglobin during frequent phlebotomies of pre-donation of autologous blood and in increasing the number of donated units but does not necessarily reduce allogeneic blood transfusions (Biesma et al, 1994; Cazenave et al, 1997; de Pree et al, 1997). However, in patients with pre-operative haemoglobin lower than 39% pre-operative erythropoietin treatment does not only facilitate predonation of autologous blood but also reduces further allogeneic blood requirements (Goodnough et al, 1997; Mott et al, 1997). Significant benefit of the erythropoietin regimen can also be expected where larger amounts of blood (5–6 units) are needed. In all cases the response of erythropoietin is dependent on iron stores and therefore additional early functional iron deficiency may further affect the response to the drug (Brugnara et al, 1993; Rutherford et al, 1994). In a recent meta-analysis Forgie et al (1998) found that pre-operative autologous donation of blood without additional erythropoietin stimulation decreases exposure to allogeneic blood but increases exposure to any transfusion (allogeneic and/or autologous). There was a direct relationship between the transfusion rate in the control group and the benefit derived from pre-operative autologous donation. On the basis of those findings, the authors suggest that other methods of decreasing blood transfusion, such as surgical technique and transfusion protocols, may be as important as pre-operative autologous donation of blood (Forgie et al, 1998).

## Alternatives to pre-deposition of autologous blood

Because of problems with pre-donation of autologous blood, there is a tendency towards replacing pre-donation with other blood conservation methods. One of them may be the extensive use of normovolaemic haemodilution, which is mainly performed after induction of anaesthesia. Although the net gain of red cells by normovolaemic haemodilution is limited (Brecher and Rosenfeld 1994; Bryson et al, 1998), normovolaemic haemodilution has been shown to be a cost-effective alternative to pre-donation in prostatectomy patients (Ness et al, 1992; Monk et al, 1998). A combination of acute normovolaemic haemodilution and pre-deposition of allogeneic blood can further decrease allogeneic blood exposure, but it increases transfusion costs and wastage. As the effectiveness of normovolaemic haemodilution is dependent on the transfusion trigger, the blood loss and the initial haemoglobin, increasing initial haemoglobin with recombinant human erythropoietin may make normovolaemic haemodilution more efficient. It has been shown that erythropoietin-supported normovolaemic haemodilution is as effective as pre-deposition of autologous blood in women undergoing primary hip replacement with regard to allogeneic blood transfusions (Stubenvoll et al, 1997). In addition, higher haemoglobin values throughout the peri-operative period may reduce the peri-operative risk, particularly in patients with cardiovascular diseases.

The contraindications for donating autologous blood are scientifically not proven but generally accepted: bacteraemia, unstable angina, critical aortic stenosis, congestive heart failure, myocardial infarction <3 months, transitory ischaemic attacks and severe uncontrolled hypertension. In patients in whom pre-deposition of autologous blood or normovolaemic haemodilution is contraindicated, pre-operative treatment with erythropoietin alone or in combination with other methods significantly reduces allogeneic transfusion requirements (Montagnac et al, 1997; Oshima et al, 1997; Rosengart et al, 1997; Sowade et al, 1997b). In elective cardiac patients erythropoietin is most useful with a peri-operative blood loss greater than 750 ml and in those with a baseline haemoglobin value less than 42% (Sowade et al, 1997b). In patients undergoing radical retropubic prostatectomy, pre-treatment with erythropoietin was as effective as predisposition of autologous blood (PAD) in reducing allogeneic blood transfusion requirements (Chun et al, 1997). The stimulation of the erythropoiesis with erythropoietin without any additional blood conservation methods resulted in a significant reduction of allogeneic transfusion in orthopaedic and cardiac surgery when compared with placebo (Anonymous, 1993; Faris et al, 1996; Sowade et al, 1997b). In general, there is a trend to lower dosages in the peri-operative setting. However, the precise role of recombinant erythropoietin in the surgical setting has not yet been established, and optimal dosage regimens have not been determined (Goldberg, 1995).

## PRE-OPERATIVE POLYCYTHAEMIA

On the one hand there is a world-wide vigorous discussion about the lowest acceptable haemoglobin; on the other hand the safe upper limit of haemoglobin is mostly ignored. Polycythaemia is rare in the peri-operative setting but, like anaemia, polycythaemia also leads to increased peri-operative morbidity and mortality and haemoglobin levels >17 g/dl in the male and >16 g/dl in the female require further diagnostic evaluation. As a consequence modifications in peri-operative treatment may become necessary. As with anaemia, polycythaemia is also a symptom of an underlying disease. Hyperviscosity becomes relevant with haematocrit levels above 60% (Well, 1975) and causes a number of complications especially thrombosis and coagulation disorders during and after surgery.

Polycythaemia vera is a neoplastic stem cell disorder characterized by excessive erythropoiesis in the presence of low endogeneous erythropoietin levels. Platelet count and white cells are often but not always elevated. The annual incidence is about 5–17 cases per million and more than 50% of the patients are older than 50 years. In the peri-operative setting patients with polycythaemia vera are rare, which may be a reason that the risk of morbidity and mortality could not be clearly defined in prospective randomized studies up until now. However, in retrospective surveys a significant higher peri-operative complication rate was found in untreated patients with polycythaemia vera when compared with treated patients (Rigby and Leavell, 1960; Wassermann and Gilbert, 1964). Almost all complications were related to the increased haemoglobin levels. Therefore, before elective surgery is performed, pre-operative treatment is essential and should be established in close co-operation with the responsible haematologist. A pre-operative reduction of haemoglobin by phlebotomies to haematocrit levels of $<45\%$ in male and 42% in female patients seems to be the most promising strategy. In the presence of extremely high haemoglobin levels and of a history of thrombotic complications the use of an automated apherese device may be more effective. Supportive therapy includes allopurinol for the prevention of secondary gout and $H_2$ blockers to prevent peptic ulcer disease. The value of anti-platelet agents such as aspirin is questionable and may cause extensive bleeding complications. In the case of emergency surgery intensive phlebotomy-accompanied volume replacement depending on the cardiovascular status should be carried out. Plateletpheresis is indicated in the case of high platelet count.

Secondary polycythaemia emerges owing to an increase of erythropoietin levels in response to hypoxia. In contrast to polycythaemia vera there is no increase of plasma volume to compensate for red cell mass (Stone et al, 1968). There is also some evidence that coagulation disorders and abnormalities in platelet function occur in patients with secondary polycythaemia (Maurer et al, 1975; Gombotz et al, 1986). In all patients with significant polycythaemia coagulation parameters should be calculated according to the circulating plasma volume. The peri-operative risk is also correlated with the increase of blood viscosity due to the haemoglobin increase, but the underlying disease seems to be the bigger issue. In a retrospective chart review of 100 patients with haemoglobin $>16$ g/dl due to chronic obstructive pulmonary disease no increase in peri-operative risk was found when compared with matched control patients (Lubarsky et al, 1991). In children with severe cyanotic heart disease pre-deposition of autologous blood was well tolerated and led to a significant reduction in allogeneic blood requirements (Gombotz et al, 1990).

Idiopathic polycythaemia is due to inappropriate secretion of erythropoietin or erythropoietin-like substances from a variety of tumours and renal abnormalities. More important for the peri-operative setting is relative polycythaemia which is relatively mild caused by contraction of the plasma volume because of diuretics or inadequate fluid intake. In the cardiovascular setting relative polycythaemia is frequently seen in middle-aged men because of stress, alcoholism, hypertension and obesity (Gaisböck syndrome). Prior to induction of anaesthesia adequate pre-load is essential to avoid drops in blood pressure and myocardial ischaemia in those patients. This is especially true for patients under acetylcholinesterase inhibitors (Burge et al, 1975).

## REFERENCES

Abels RI (1992) Use of recombinant human erythropoietin in the treatment of anemia in patients who have cancer. *Seminars in Oncology* **19:** 29–35.

Ania BJ, Suman VJ, Fairbanks VF et al (1997) Incidence of anemia in older people: an epidemiologic study in a well defined population. *Journal of the American Geriatrics Society* **45:** 825–831.

Anonymous (1968) World Health Organization. Nutritional anaemias. Report of a WHO Scientific Group. *Technical Report Series* No. 405, Geneva.

Anonymous (1993) Effectiveness of perioperative recombinant human erythropoietin in elective hip replacement. Canadian Orthopedic Perioperative Erythropoietin Study Group. *Lancet* **341:** 1227–1232.

Audet AM, Goodnough LT & Parvin CA (1996) Evaluating the appropriateness of red blood cell transfusions: the limitations of retrospective medical record reviews. *International Journal of Quality Health Care* **8:** 41–49.

Axelrod FB, Pepkowitz SH & Goldfinger D (1989) Establishment of a schedule of optimal preoperative collection of autologous blood. *Transfusion* **29:** 677–680.

Biesma DH, Kraaijenhagen RJ, Poortman J et al (1992) The effect of oral iron supplementation on erythropoiesis in autologous blood donors. *Transfusion* **32:** 162–165.

Biesma DH, Marx JJ, Kraaijenhagen RJ et al (1994) Lower homologous blood requirement in autologous blood donors after treatment with recombinant human erythropoietin. *Lancet* **344:** 367–370.

Brecher ME & Rosenfeld M (1994) Mathematical and computer modeling of acute normovolemic hemodilution. *Transfusion* **34:** 176–179.

Brugnara C, Chambers LA, Malynn E et al (1993) Red blood cell regeneration induced by subcutaneous recombinant erythropoietin: iron-deficient erythropoiesis in iron-replete subjects. *Blood* **81:** 956–964.

Bryson GL, Laupacis A & Wells GA (1998) Does acute normovolemic hemodilution reduce perioperative allogeneic transfusion? A meta-analysis. The International Study of Perioperative Transfusion. *Anesthesia and Analgesia* **86:** 9–15.

Burge PS, Johnson WS & Prankerd TAJ (1975) Morbidity and mortality in pseudopolycythemia. *Lancet* **2:** 1266–1270.

*Carson JL, Poses RM, Spence RK & Bonavita G (1988) Severity of anaemia and operative mortality and morbidity. *Lancet* **1:** 727–729.

*Carson JL, Duff A, Poses RM et al (1996) Effect of anaemia and cardiovascular disease on surgical mortality and morbidity. *Lancet* **348:** 1055–1060.

Carson JL, Duff A, Berlin JA et al (1998) Perioperative blood transfusion and postoperative mortality. *Journal of the American Medical Association* **279:** 199–205.

Cazenave JP, Irrmann C, Waller C et al (1997) Epoetin alfa facilitates presurgical autologous blood donation in non-anaemic patients scheduled for orthopaedic or cardiovascular surgery. *European Journal of Anaesthesiology* **14:** 432–442.

*Cazzola M, Mercuriali F & Brugnara C (1997) Use of recombinant human erythropoietin outside the setting of uremia. *Blood* **89:** 4248–4267.

Chun TY, Martin S & Lepor H (1997) Preoperative recombinant human erythropoietin injection versus preoperative autologous blood donation in patients undergoing radical retropubic prostatectomy. *Urology* **50:** 727–732.

Crystal GJ, Rooney MW & Salem MR (1988) Myocardial blood flow and oxygen consumption during isovolemic hemodilution alone and in combination with adenosine-induced controlled hypotension. *Anesthesia and Analgesia* **67:** 539–547.

Dong WK, Bledsoe SW, Chadwick HS et al (1986) Electrical correlates of brain injury resulting from severe hypotension and hemodilution in monkeys. *Anesthesiology* **65:** 617–625.

Drueke TB, Barany P, Cazzola M et al (1997) Management of iron deficiency in renal anemia: guidelines for the optimal therapeutic approach in erythropoietin-treated patients. *Clinical Nephrology* **48:** 1–8.

van Dyck MJ, Baele PL, Leclercq P et al (1994) Autologous blood donation before myocardial revascularization: a Holter-electrocardiographic analysis. *Journal of Cardiothoracic and Vascular Anesthesia* **8:** 162–167.

Eschbach JW, Kelly MR, Haley NR et al (1989) Treatment of the anemia of progressive renal failure with recombinant human erythropoietin. *New England Journal of Medicine* **321:** 158–163.

Etchason J, Petz L, Keeler E et al (1995) The cost effectiveness of preoperative autologous blood donations. *New England Journal of Medicine* **332:** 719–724.

Fang WC, Helm RE, Krieger KH et al (1997) Impact of minimum hematocrit during cardiopulmonary bypass on mortality in patients undergoing coronary artery surgery. *Circulation* **96 (supplement II):** II194–II199.

Faris PM, Ritter MA & Abels RI (1996) The effects of recombinant human erythropoietin on perioperative transfusion requirements in patients having a major orthopaedic operation. The American Erythropoietin Study Group. *Journal of Bone and Joint Surgery, American Volume* **78:** 62–72.

Ferguson BJ, Skikne BS, Simpson KM et al (1992) Serum transferrin receptor distinguishes the anemia of chronic disease from iron deficiency anemia. *Journal of Laboratory and Clinical Medicine* **119:** 385–390.

Fitzgerald RD, Martin MC, Dietz GE et al (1997) Transfusing red blood cells stored in citrate phosphate dextrose adenine-1 for 28 days fails to improve tissue oxygenation in rats. *Critical Care Medicine* **25:** 726–732.

Forgie MA, Wells PS, Laupacis A & Fergusson D (1998) Preoperative autologous donation decreases allogeneic transfusion but increases exposure to all red blood cell transfusion: results of a meta-analysis. International Study of Perioperative Transfusion (ISPOT) Investigators. *Archives of Internal Medicine* **158:** 610–616.

Friedman BA, Oberman HA, Chadwick AR & Kingdon KI (1976) The maximum surgical blood order schedule and surgical blood use in the United States. *Transfusion* **16:** 380–387.

Gagnon DR, Zhang TJ, Brand FN & Kannel WB (1994) Hematocrit and the risk of cardiovascular disease—the Framingham study: a 34-year follow-up. *American Heart Journal* **127:** 674–682.

Goh M, Kleer CG, Kielczewski P et al (1997) Autologous blood donation prior to anatomical radical retropubic prostatectomy: is it necessary? *Urology* **49:** 569–573.

Goldberg MA (1995) Erythropoiesis, erythropoietin, and iron metabolism in elective surgery: preoperative strategies for avoiding allogeneic blood exposure. *American Journal of Surgery* **170:** 37S–43S.

Goldman M, Remy PS, Trepanier A & Decary F (1997) Autologous donation error rates in Canada. *Transfusion* **37:** 523–527.

Gombotz H & Kulier A (1995) Reduktion des Fremdblutverbrauchs in der operativen Medizin. *Anaesthesist* **44:** 191–218.

Gombotz H, Metzler H & Hiotakis K (1986) Antithrombin-III-Verhalten bei offenen Herzoperationen im Säuglings- und Kleinkindesalter. *Anästhesie, Intensivemedizin, Notfallmedizin* **21:** 9–12.

Gombotz H, Stein J, Suppan CH et al (1990) Hemodynamic alterations during autologous blood donation for children in severe cyanotic heart disease. *Anesthesiology* **73:** A1118 (abstract).

*Goodnough LT, Monk TG & Andriole GL (1997) Erythropoietin therapy. *New England Journal of Medicine* **336:** 933–938.

Hackmann T, Steward DJ & Sheps SB (1991) Anemia in pediatric day-surgery patients: prevalence and detection. *Anesthesiology* **75:** 27–31.

Harthoorn LE, Lindemans J & Langenhuijsen MM (1998) Zinc protoporphyrin as screening test in female blood donors. *Clinical Chemistry* **44:** 800–804.

Hebert PC, Wells G, Tweeddale M et al (1997) Does transfusion practice affect mortality in critically ill patients? Transfusion Requirements in Critical Care (TRICC) Investigators and the Canadian Critical Care Trials Group. *American Journal of Respiratory and Critical Care Medicine* **155:** 1618–1623.

Hebert PC, Wells G, Martin C et al (1998) A Canadian survey of transfusion practices in critically ill patients. Transfusion Requirements in Critical Care Investigators and the Canadian Critical Care Trials Group. *Critical Care Medicine* **26:** 482–487.

Helm RE, Rosengart TK, Gomez M et al (1998) Comprehensive multimodality blood conservation: 100 consecutive CABG operations without transfusion. *Annals of Thoracic Surgery* **65:** 125–136.

Hillyer CD, Hart KK, Lackey DA et al (1994) Comparable safety of blood collection in 'high-risk' autologous donors versus non-high-risk autologous and directed donors in a hospital setting. *American Journal of Clinical Pathology* **102:** 275–277.

van Iterson M, van der Waart FJ, Erdmann W & Trouwborst A (1995) Systemic haemodynamics and oxygenation during haemodilution in children. *Lancet* **346:** 1127–1129.

Jan KM & Chien S (1977) Effect of hematocrit variations on coronary hemodynamics and oxygen utilization. *American Journal of Physiology* **233:** H106–H113.

Kanter MH, Van MD, Anders KH et al (1996) Preoperative autologous blood donations before elective hysterectomy. *Journal of the American Medical Association* **276:** 798–801.

Kasper SM, Baumann M, Radbruch L et al (1997a) A pilot study of continuous ambulatory electrocardiography in patients donating blood for autologous use in elective coronary artery bypass grafting. *Transfusion* **37:** 829–835.

Kasper SM, Gerlich W & Buzello W (1997b) Preoperative red cell production in patients undergoing weekly autologous blood donation. *Transfusion* **37:** 1058–1062.

Kulier AH, Gombotz H, Fuchs G et al (1993) Subcutaneous recombinant human erythropoietin and autologous blood donation before coronary artery bypass surgery. *Anesthesia and Analgesia* **76:** 102–106.

Larocque BJ, Gilbert K & Brien WF (1997) A point score system for predicting the likelihood of blood transfusion after hip or knee arthroplasty. *Transfusion* **37:** 463–467.

Larsen N, Foyt M & Marengo-Rowe A (1994) Late donation of autologous units increases allogenic transfusion requirements. *Transfusion* **35:** S96 (abstract).

Lorentz A, Eckardt KU, Osswald PM & Duchow JR (1992) Erythropoietin levels in patients depositing autologous blood in short intervals. *Annals of Hematology* **64:** 281–285.

Lubarsky DA, Gallagher CJ & Berend JL (1991) Secondary polycythemia does not increase the risk of perioperative hemorrhagic or thrombotic complications. *Journal of Clinical Anesthesia* **3:** 99–103.

McPhee SJ (1982) The evaluation of anaemia. *Western Journal of Medicine* **137:** 253–257.

McVay PA, Andrews A, Hoag MS et al (1990) Moderate and severe reactions during autologous blood donations are no more frequent than during homologous blood donations. *Vox Sanguinis* **59:** 70–72.

Marik PE & Sibbald WJ (1993) Effect of stored-blood transfusion on oxygen delivery in patients with sepsis. *Journal of the American Medical Association* **269:** 3024–3029.

Maurer HM, McCue CM, Robertson LW & Haggins JC (1975) Correction of platelet dysfunction and bleeding in cyanotic congenital heart disease by simple red volume reduction. *American Journal of Cardiology* **35:** 831–835.

Means RT & Krantz SB (1992) Progress in understanding the pathogenesis of the anemia of chronic disease. *Blood* **80:** 1639–1647.

*Mercuriali F & Intaglietta M (1996) Proposal of an algorithm to help the choice of the best transfusion strategy. *Current Medical Research Opinion* **13:** 465–478.

Mercuriali F & Inghilleri G (in press) Management of perioperative anaemia. *British Journal of Anaesthesia* **81 (supplement 1):** 56–61.

Mercuriali F, Inghilleri G, Biffi E et al (1997) Comparison between intravenous and subcutaneous recombinant human erythropoietin (Epoetin alfa) administration in presurgical autologous blood donation in anemic rheumatoid arthritis patients undergoing major orthopedic surgery. *Vox Sanguinis* **72:** 93–100.

Messmer K (1981) Compensatory mechanisms for acute dilutional anemia. *Bibliographia Haematologica* **47:** 31–42.

Messmer K, Kreimeier U & Intaglietta M (1986) Present state of intentional hemodilution. *European Surgical Research* **18:** 254–263.

Monk TG, Goodnough LT, Brecher ME et al (1998) Acute normovolemic hemodilution can replace preoperative autologous blood donation as a standard of care for autologous blood procurement in radical prostatectomy. *Anesthesia and Analgesia* **85:** 953–958.

Montagnac R, Ebikili B & Schillinger F (1997) Recombinant human erythropoietin (epoetin) and autologous blood transfusion in chronic hemodialysis. Apropos of 2 cases. *Nephrologie* **18:** 23–26.

Mott LS, Bechinski J & Jones MJ (1997) Autologous blood collection in anemic patients using low-dose erythropoietin therapy. *Journal of the National Medical Association* **89:** 381–384.

Nelson AH, Fleisher LA & Rosenbaum SH (1993) Relationship between postoperative anemia and cardiac morbidity in high-risk vascular patients in the intensive care unit. *Critical Care Medicine* **21:** 860–866.

Ness PM, Bourke DL & Walsh PC (1992) A randomized trial of perioperative hemodilution versus transfusion of preoperatively deposited autologous blood in elective surgery. *Transfusion* **32:** 226–230.

Nuttall GA, Santrach PJ, Oliver WC et al (1996) The predictors of red cell transfusions in total hip arthroplasties. *Transfusion* **36:** 144–149.

Oshima N, Kiyama H & Imazeki T (1997) Combined erythropoietin and aprotinin use for blood conservation in elderly coronary bypass patients. *Kyobu Geka* **50:** 707–710.

Pincus T, Olsen NJ, Russell IJ et al (1990) Multicenter study of recombinant human erythropoietin in correction of anemia in rheumatoid arthritis. *American Journal of Medicine* **89:** 161–168.

Plewes JL & Farhi LE (1985) Cardiovascular responses to hemodilution and controlled hypotension in the dog. *Anesthesiology* **62:** 149–154.

Popovsky MA, Whitaker B & Arnold NL (1995) Severe outcomes of allogeneic and autologous blood donation: frequency and characterization. *Transfusion* **35:** 734–737.

Posch U, Stubenvoll E, Pätzold D et al (1994) Zinkprotoporphyrin als Verlaufsparameter für den Eisenstoffwechsel im Rahmen der präoperativen Eigenblutspende. In Mempel W, Schwarzfischer G & Mempel Ch (eds) *Eigenbluttransfusion heute*, pp 185–190. Munich: Sympomed.

de Pree C, Mermillod B, Hoffmeyer P & Beris P (1997) Recombinant human erythropoietin as adjuvant treatment for autologous blood donation in elective surgery with large blood needs (⩾5 units): a randomized study. *Transfusion* **37:** 708–714.

Rady MY, Ryan T & Starr NJ (1998) Perioperative determinants of morbidity and mortality in elderly patients undergoing cardiac surgery. *Critical Care Medicine* **26:** 225–235.

von Restorff W, Höfling B, Holtz J & Bassenge E (1975) Effect of increased blood fluidity through hemodilution on general circulation at rest and during exercise in dogs. *Pflugers Archiv* **357:** 25–34.

Rigby PG & Leavell BS (1960) Polycythemia vera: a review of fifty cases with emphasis on risk of surgery. *Archives of Internal Medicine* **106:** 622–627.

Rosengart TK, Helm RE, DeBois WJ et al (1997) Open heart operations without transfusion using a multimodality blood conservation strategy in 50 Jehovah's Witness patients: implications for a 'bloodless' surgical technique. *Journal of the American College of Surgery* **184:** 618–629.

Rutherford CJ, Schneider TJ, Dempsey H et al (1994) Efficacy of different dosing regimens for recombinant human erythropoietin in a simulated perisurgical setting: the importance of iron availability in optimizing response. *American Journal of Medicine* **96:** 139–145.

Skikne BS & Cook JD (1992) Effect of enhanced erythropoiesis on iron absorption. *Journal of Laboratory and Clinical Medicine* **120:** 746–751.

Sowade O, Sowade B, Brilla K et al (1997a) Kinetics of reticulocyte maturity fractions and indices and iron status during therapy with epoetin beta (recombinant human erythropoietin) in cardiac surgery patients. *American Journal of Hematology* **55:** 89–96.

Sowade O, Warnke H, Scigalla P et al (1997b) Avoidance of allogeneic blood transfusions by treatment with epoetin beta (recombinant human erythropoietin) in patients undergoing open-heart surgery. *Blood* **89:** 411–418.

*Spahn DR, Leone BJ, Reves JG & Pasch T (1994) Cardiovascular and coronary physiology of acute isovolemic hemodilution: a review of nonoxygen-carrying and oxygen-carrying solutions. *Anesthesia and Analgesia* **78:** 1000–1021.

Spahn DR, Schmid ER, Seifert B & Pasch T (1996a) Hemodilution tolerance in patients with coronary artery disease who are receiving chronic beta-adrenergic blocker therapy. *Anesthesia and Analgesia* **82:** 687–694.

Spahn DR, Zollinger A, Schlumpf RB et al (1996b) Hemodilution tolerance in elderly patients without known cardiac disease. *Anesthesia and Analgesia* **82:** 681–686.

Spence RK, Carson JA, Poses R et al (1990) Elective surgery without tranfusion: influence of preoperative hemoglobin level and blood loss on mortality. *American Journal of Surgery* **159:** 320–324.

Spiess BD, Sassetti R, McCarthy RJ et al (1992) Autologous blood donation: hemodynamics in a high-risk patient population. *Transfusion* **32:** 17–22.

Spivak JL (1994) Cancer-related anemia: its causes and characteristics. *Seminars in Oncology* **21:** 3–8.

Stone HO, Thompson AK Jr & Schmiedt-Nielson K (1968) Influence of erythrocytes on blood viscosity. *American Journal of Physiology* **214:** 913–918.

Stover EP, Siegel L, Parks R et al (1998) Variability in transfusion practice for coronary artery bypass surgery persists despite national consensus guidelines. *Anesthesiology* **88:** 327–333.

Stubenvoll E, Gries M, Gombotz H et al (1997) Comparison of EPO-supported haemodilution with predonation of autologous blood for total hip replacement. *British Journal of Anaesthesia* **78:** 65.

Sunder-Plassmann L, Kessler M & Jesch F (1975) Acute normovolemic hemodilution: changes in tissue oxygen supply and hemoglobin–oxygen affinity. *Bibliographica Haematologica* **41:** 44–53.

Toy P, Ahn DK & Bacchetti P (1994) When should the first of two donations be made? *Transfusion* **34:** S54 (abstract).

Viele MK & Weiskopf RB (1994) What can we learn about the need for transfusion from patients who refuse blood? The experience with Jehovah's Witnesses. *Transfusion* **34:** 396–401.

Vreugdenhil G, Baltus CA, Van EH & Swaak AJ (1990) Anaemia of chronic disease: diagnostic significance of erythrocyte and serological parameters in iron deficient rheumatoid arthritis patients. *British Journal of Rheumatology* **29:** 105–110.

Vreugdenhil G, Lowenberg B, Van EH & Swaak AJ (1992) Tumor necrosis factor alpha is associated with disease activity and the degree of anemia in patients with rheumatoid arthritis. *European Journal of Clinical Investigation* **22:** 488–493.

Wassermann LR & Gilbert HS (1964) Surgical bleeding in polycytemia vera. *Annals of the New York Academy of Sciences* **115:** 122–138.

Weiskopf RB, Viele MK, Feiner J et al (1998) Human cardiovascular and metabolic response to acute, severe isovolemic anemia. *Journal of the American Medical Association* **279:** 217–221.

Well R (1975) Syndromes of hyperviscosity. *New England Journal of Medicine* **283:** 183–186.

# 10

# Scores, scoring and outcome: correlation between pre-operative assessment and post-operative morbidity and mortality of non-hospitalized and hospitalized patients

PETER M. OSSWALD MD

Director

OLAV SWARS MD

Assistant resident

PATRICIA LEUFKE

Assistant

*Institut für Anaesthesiologie und operative Intensivmedizin, Klinikum Stadt Hanau, Leimenstr. 20, 63450 Hanau, Germany*

Anaesthetists are occupied with the possibility of complications during the peri-operative period. All previously published proposals have attempted to estimate the pre-operative state of the patient in order to be able to judge the risk of the impending anaesthetic treatment more reliably. In this chapter we describe the predictive value of the most common anaesthetic classification systems. The prediction of the ASA grade, the Goldman cardiac risk index, the Mannheim checklist and the Munich checklist for peri-operative complications are analysed. Furthermore, we give an overview of the extensive literature of the risk classification in anaesthesia in the different medicine compartments with a special view on ambulatory patients.

**Key words:** scores; outcome; peri-operative anaesthetic risk; risk classification; ambulatory anaesthesia.

## DEVELOPMENT AND DESCRIPTION OF THE PROBLEM

Medical risk can be defined as the danger that occurs when medical procedures fail. The risk is the theoretical, ex ante presupposed danger of treatment failure. A complication on the other hand is a difficulty or setback that appears in an individual case and in which the risk has become tangible

*Baillière's Clinical Anaesthesiology*—
Vol. 12, No. 3, September 1998
ISBN 0–7020–2536–4
0950–3501/98/030471 + 13 $12.00/00

and, to the extent to which it is not controlled, has already taken effect. Peri-operative complications depend on the urgency of the operation and the health status of the patient. Serious cardiovascular disturbances, age, site of the operation and the experience of the surgeon and anaesthetist and also other environmental and staff circumstances play an important role. An essential factor for a complication-free anaesthesia and peri-operative phase is the pre-operative examination and the recognition of potential risk factors by an experienced anaesthetist.

If a reduction of the anaesthetic risk is to be achieved by therapeutic intervention, systematic methods for the early discovery of risks caused by illness are indispensable. Many of these methods rely upon the processing of scales and scores. For example, Virginia Apgar developed the internationally acknowledged Apgar score for the evaluation of a newborn's well-being.

Anaesthetists have been occupied with the possibility of risk analysis for more than 40 years. Although significant progress has been made in this field, the problem has as yet not been solved. All previously published proposals have attempted to estimate the pre-operative state of the patient in order to be able to judge the risk of the impending anaesthetic treatment more reliably.

## AMERICAN SOCIETY OF ANAESTHESIOLOGISTS CLASSIFICATION

In 1941 a Commission of the American Society of Anesthetists (ASA) worked out a system of classification that ranked the pre-operative state of the patient in four groups. In 1961 they extended this to five groups. Two years later, the ASA officially recommended the system for pre-operative risk classification. The ASA 1963 classified a new scheme of the health state (ASA Physical Status) and confirmed five physical states:

ASA 1, normal healthy patient
ASA 2, patient with light systematic disease
ASA 3, patient with serious systematic disease and performance reduction
ASA 4, patient with most serious systematic disease and constant life threat
ASA 5, moribund patient who probably will not survive the next 24 hours

In emergency operations, an 'E' ('emergency') is put in front of the ASA class. The ASA classification has achieved worldwide recognition because of its simplicity, transparency and comparability.

However, a consideration of this scheme makes it clear that it enables only an inadequate judgement because the subjective assessment of the user is allowed too much influence and neither significant secondary illness nor the effects of the surgery itself are taken into account. Even though the anaesthesiological mortality is not to be seen as a reliable preview through risk classification measurement, the ASA classification has carried out a good job as a standard scoring system with good results.

Although its introduction is considered to have been an important milestone on the way to pre-operative risk classification, the criticism of this system has never stopped. All comprehensive attempts at risk judgement in anaesthetics begin with the description of fatal accidents, then retrospectively examine intraoperative mortality and then prospectively examine the peri-operative morbidity and mortality of the operated patient. This reveals ways that aim to improve the evaluation of risk, i.e. more security for the patient. The cause of the unconvincing results of such scoring systems is above all that such systems often rely on non-objective criteria and leave room for the doctor's own discretion about the classification of the patient's risk grouping. Misjudgement is unavoidable.

Several trials of risk assessment in anaesthesia have been performed upon researched intraoperative cases of death, which contain the retrospective description of cases ending in death and the prospective research of perioperative morbidity and mortality of patients. This system show ways which until today have been followed to calculate the risk in the sense of increased security of our patients. Even though retrospective examinations have proven their value in the past, there is still a need to do further prospective research in different categories of age, illness and specific operation to analyse the risk of the patient expecting an operation as precisely as possible or even to eliminate the risk. There is no doubt that the ASA classification lacks precision. Referring to documentations of 10 hypothetical patients Owens et al (1978) could only find a very vague confirmation of the ASA classification. In particular, age, adiposis, a pre-myocardial infarction and anaemia were judged controversially. The sort of operation also cannot be judged, as well as intubation complications, transfusion complications or malignant hyperthermia. Even though lacking precision, the ASA classification has proven useful not only in the USA but also in Europe because of its simplicity, transparency and comparability. Differences in judgement from one patient to another probably exist from hospital to hospital. Using the ASA classification is already very helpful in the authors' institution, because it enables comparison of the disease severity for the anaesthetist as well as for the surgeon and there can be either an expansion or a reduction of the operative procedure.

## CARDIAC RISK INDEX

The multifactorial cardiac risk index (CRI) for non-cardiac surgical operations used in the prospective study by Goldman et al of 1001 patients more than 40 years of age draws attention to the pre-operative assessment especially of the cardiovascular system.

On the basis of research on 1001 patients, Goldman et al (1977) developed a multifactorial CRI for non-cardiac surgical operations. The risk factors in Table 1 were distinguished.

In 1977 Goldman et al published a study of the cardiac risk in non-cardiac surgery. They used risk factors that correlated closely with serious post-operative outcome. Because of the high percentage of secondary

**Table 1.** Risk factors.

| | | |
|---|---|---|
| 1. | Pre-operative third heartbeat or jugular venal pulsation | 11 points |
| 2. | Myocardial attack less than 6 months ago | 10 points |
| 3. | No sinus rhythm or supraventricular extrasystolic | 7 points |
| 4. | More than five ventricular extrasystolics pre-operative | 7 points |
| 5. | Age over 70 years | 5 points |
| 6. | Aorta operation | 4 points |
| 7. | Aorta valve stenosis | 3 points |
| 8. | Emergency operation | 4 points |
| 9. | Bad general state of health | 3 points |
| CRI | | |
| Class 1 | 0–5 points | |
| Class 2 | 6–12 points | |
| Class 3 | 13–25 points | |
| Class 4 | >25 points | |

cardiovascular disease and complications, this essay is considered a useful contribution to the search for a reliable method of pre-operative risk classification. Also, the essay published by Goldman and his colleagues was the first real attempt to analyse the risks. With the help of logistic discrimination analysis, the high reliability in the prediction of the complications that occurred could be verified. Owen et al (1978) discovered, in very widespread research, that this scoring of surgical procedures could not to be used for the aorta abdominalis. Detsky et al (1986) described a multifactorial CRI that can be used to assess patients undergoing non-cardiac surgery. The index is a modified version of the Goldman index and was prospectively validated on 455 patients. They present a Bayesian approach to assessing cardiac risks by converting average risks for patients undergoing particular surgical procedures (pre-test probabilities) to average risks by converting average risks with each index score (post-test probabilities). In particular, silent angina enters into the classification as an increase of points. A simple nomogram is presented for performing such a calculation.

## MANNHEIM CHECKLIST

With the so-called Mannheim checklist, Lutz (1972) were able to introduce a new classification system. In this scoring system the necessity to operate, type of operation, the duration of the operation, weight, blood pressure, heart performance, electrocardiogram (ECG), breathing and laboratory values are rated with points. The parameter which is built upon a scale of descending quality ensures an apportionment of 0–16 points (0 points normal, 16 points widest deviation).

The Mannheim checklist allows a much better estimate of the presenting illness of the surgical patient because it predominantly relies on objective criteria. In the evaluation of intra- and post-operative complications, a gradual increase in the complications and fatal accidents could be identified with increasing risk group. The advantage of the Mannheim checklist is the precision of the correlation of the increasing scores with the increasing seriousness of the disease and of the operation. The disadvantage is the poor transparency of the scores, the complexity and the failing comparison with the ASA classification.

Five risk groups are formed out of the sum of the points.

Risk group 1, 0–2 points
Risk group 2, 3–5 points
Risk group 3, 6–10 points
Risk group 4, 11–20 points
Risk group 5, >20 points

The Mannheim checklist allows an exact prognosis but because it is complicated to use and because of its relatively poor transparency it has not found widespread application.

## THE MUNICH CHECKLIST

The so-called Munich risk checklist published by Peter et al (1980) uses three risk classes. Age, site of operation, cardiac performance, cardiac rhythm, circulation, pulmonary function, laboratory values, anaesthetic duration and urgency of operation are evaluated. The Munich risk checklist allows an exact prognosis and because it uses only three risk classes it provides the advantage of a better overview. The missing comparability with the ASA score is a slight disadvantage.

Peter et al (1980) worked out a checklist that to a large extent developed upon the Mannheim checklist. The main difference from the Mannheim risk score is that instead of a geometric increasing loading there is an arithmetic judgement of the findings and that no longer five but three groups are distinguished. The concentration of the patients into three groups was done in order to increase the correlation with the rate of complication. It has the advantage of being comprehensive but the scores are nonetheless not transparent and the three risk classes are not comparable with the five ASA classes. It is also not widely used.

## RISK CLASSIFICATION

From an overview of the extensive literature (Table 2) it becomes clear that, with regard to the validation and application of scoring systems, only in a few cases do the authors also make statements about sensitivity or specificity. Often they describe only the use and the weight of the score system with regard to better estimation and risk reduction in general.

The number of examined patients varies enormously, the statements are concerned for the greatest part with the identification of a good correlation between the measured risk and their correlations. Precise statements about mortality and morbidity can only be given as percentages. No distinctions are made about when such examinations should be carried out in general

**Table 2.** Overview of literature on risk classification.

| Section | Theme | Reference | Patients *N* | Main risk |
|---|---|---|---|---|
| General surgery | Lung complications after laparatomy | Hall et al (1991) | 1000 | ASA status |
| General surgery | ASA score | Menke et al (1993) | 2248 | ASA status |
| General surgery | ASA–Goldmann–preview peri-operative mortality | Prause et al (1997a) | 16 227 | ASA status, score |
| General surgery | Score for preview peri-operative bronchospasm | Harada (1995) | 32 | Bronchial asthma |
| General surgery–cardiac surgery | Preview post-operative cardiac ischaemic state | Howell et al (1997) | 183 | Pre-operative ischaemia, high pressure |
| Anaesthesiology | Pre-operative ambulance, Graz | Prause (1997b) | 75 000 | Cardiovascular nephrological disease, ASA status |
| Anaesthesiology | Preview–peri-operative outcome | Forrest (1992) | 17 201 | 17 and 9 Risil Text |
| Internal medicine | Smoker–lung function | Browner et al (1992) | 6347 | Smoking, lung |
| Anaesthesiology–general surgery | Death in anaesthesia in Finland | Tikkanen et al (1995) | 325 585 | |

surgery, emergency surgery, thorax or vascular surgery or in other areas. The situation alone of the published studies shows the great need for a reliable risk estimation.

## General surgery on hospitalized patients

In a study of 16 227 patients, Prause et al (1997b) examined the correlation of peri-operative mortality with the categories of the ASA classification and the categories of the Goldman scoring system. Of all patients studied, 215 died within the first 4 weeks after the operation. Both scoring systems which were examined correlated well with regard to the size of the risk estimation and with post-operative mortality. The combination of both score systems gave an even better prognosis of the post-operative mortality. A study by Menke et al (1993) is concerned with a similar question. The prognosis of the peri-operative morbidity and mortality in connection with the ASA classification was also examined. In 2248 patients, it was shown that post-operative morbidity ranged from 3.9% in the ASA 1 group to 33.7% in the ASA 4 group. Not one patient in the ASA 1 group died, whereas 7.2% died of those who before the operation were registered in the ASA 4 group. A clear correlation between the pre-operative rating of the ASA classification and the peri-operative morbidity and mortality is also demonstrated in this study. Furthermore, a strong link between the risk and the duration of the hospitalization and of intensive care could also be seen.

In 1992 Forrest studied the prognosis of the post-operative outcome with independent predictors in 17 201 patients. They were able to evaluate 17 significant predictors (history of ventricular arrhythmia, hypertension, cardiac failure, myocardial ischaemia, myocardial infarction less than or equal to 1 year, myocardial infarction greater than 1 year, smoking, ASA physical status, age, cardiovascular, thoracic, abdominal eye–ear–nose–throat, endocrine, neurological, musculoskeletal or gynaecological surgery and the study anaesthetics) for 10 serious cardiovascular incidents and nine significant predictors (history of cardiac failure, myocardial ischaemia, chronic obstructive pulmonary disease, obesity, smoking, male gender, ASA physical status, abdominal surgery and the study anaesthetics) for four serious respiratory complications. Also, in this work, a significant connection between the level of the ASA classification and the occurrence of peri-operative complications could be demonstrated.

Chijiiwa et al (1996) examined the correlation of pre-operative ASA status and the occurrence of post-operative complications in 69 pancreatico-duodenotomy patients. The authors did not find a direct correlation between the post-operative complications and the ASA status. However, the study was more concerned with the long-term outcome.

Hall et al (1996) examined the influence of age and the pre-operative ASA classification on the occurrence of complications in 2570 patients undergoing abdominal surgery. The results of this study showed that the ASA classification together with the age of the patient can be used as important predictors of the risk of peri-operative complications. Exact statements as to the specifics, significance and sensitivity were not presented. Martin (1992) examined the requirements of a reasonable peri-operative management of old patients. One can summarize that an intensive pre-operative diagnosis of the accompanying ailment increases the probability of accurate forecast of peri-operative complications. Van der Merwe et al (1992) examined the influence of pre-operative management of patients with coronary heart disease; the prognosis of post-operative complications through pre-operative diagnosis was tested. This study also demonstrated that the quality and the range of the pre-operative findings correlated with the prognosis of complications. Hennein et al (1994) searched for predictors of peri-operative complications in patients with an innate cardiac defect. Also in this study the ASA classification allowed a prognosis of the risk of peri-operative complication.

Mangano et al (1992) examined the long-term outcome of 444 patients with chronic cardiovascular disease. This group of patients showed a significantly higher incidence of peri-operative complication. Patients with acute cardiac ischaemia had the highest risk. O'Kelly et al (1992) were able to determine the probability of the appearance of ventricular rhythm disturbances with the help of predictors. As a result one can say that half of the so-called high-risk patients developed peri-operative ventricular rhythm disturbances. They showed that invasive monitoring did not lead to an increased risk of serious ventricular rhythm disturbance. Forrest described adrial fibrillation as an important risk-factor. Masutani et al (1992) studied ECGs peri-operatively and the prognosis of ECG fluctuations. Several factors were found which increased the incidence of dysrhythmias: age, type of operation, intraoperative rhythm disturbance, loss of blood, duration of operation, adjusted arterial blood pressure. Also, the ASA classification and the Goldman score increased the prognosis of ventricular rhythm disturbance in the peri-operative phase. Howell et al (1997) looked for predictors of post-operative cardiac ischaemia in 183 patients. Arterial hypertension was of central interest in the study. It could be demonstrated that the risk of peri-operative cardiac ischaemia was directly correlated with the height of the arterial blood pressure. Hall et al (1991) examined the predictability of pulmonary complications in 1000 patients undergoing laparotomy. It was also shown here that the pre-operative risk rating according to the ASA classification correlated well with the incidence of pulmonary complication. A combination of the ASA rating with the age of the patient was able to improve the prognosis itself. In a retrospective study, Howell et al (1997) studied the connection between arterial blood pressure and cardiovascular complication in 76 patients who died after the operation. No connection was found between the height of systolic or diastolic blood pressure and patient mortality. The studies offer a realization of pivotal facts, determining the preview in a substantial way. Substantial criteria are lung function, age, sex, being a smoker and cardiac failure.

## General surgery on non-hospitalized patients

Kvalsvik et al (1996) studied the selection of patients for outpatient surgery and/or anaesthesia. They concluded that it is necessary to create systems in outpatient clinics which are able to evaluate patients with a higher anaesthetic risk. According to Kvalsvik et al the vast majority of patients with ASA 3 rating and even a large number of patients rated ASA 4 operatively can be safely operated on in an outpatient surgery unit. Duncan et al (1992) examined the relationship in 6914 patients between various events in the peri-operative phase in the light of the pre-operative diagnosis. A correlation between the pre-operative state of health and the incidence of complications could be demonstrated. Heino et al (1992) examined the outcome of outpatient surgery in 597 patients. The reasons for and the frequency of a doctor's visit after the operation were retrospectively examined. In summary it can be said that no ambulatory patient died and that no serious complication occurred. Of the patients studied, 92% were satisfied with surgery and anaesthesia. The most frequent reasons for post-operative consultation were pain, minor bleeding and wound infection. Warner et al (1993) looked for the most frequent causes of morbidity and mortality in outpatient surgery. Data on 38 598 patients were evaluated. Thirty-three patients had serious complications and four patients died, two as a result of a heart attack and two as a result of a traffic accident. Of the 33 patients with serious complications, 14 had myocardial attacks, seven had dysfunctions of the central nervous system, five had pulmonary embolisms and five had respiratory complications. All in all, the authors rate the total rate of mortality and morbidity as minimal. Cassidy et al (1996) examined the pre-operative behaviour and the management of anaesthetized outpatients. Cassidy et al also considered that pre-operative estimation of risk is worthwhile and they developed a catalogue in which the pre-operative treatment requirements are listed. An exact internal–surgical–anaesthesiological patient history, physical examination and necessary diagnosis based on apparative systems like ECG, X-ray, etc. are required as a guide.

## Anaesthesiology

Goldman et al (1977) published a study in which they presented an index for the assessment of cardiac risk in operations with the exception of heart–thorax surgery. One thousand patients over the age of 40 years were examined. Goldman et al were able to determine nine independent risk factors which correlated with the frequency of cardiac incidents. Tikkanen et al (1995) examined the total rate of mortality after operations in Finnish patients. In all 325 585 patients were studied: 570 patients died, 22 of which were caused by surgery and five deaths had an anaesthesiological cause. Davies (1994) compared a pre-operative risk rating produced by a computer program with the evaluation of the anaesthesiologist. The computer had a modified version of the ASA classification. Male patients between the ages of 30 and 50 years were considered. Twenty-seven anaesthetists made estimations of the pre-operative risk. A corresponding risk estimation was made by the computer program. Eleven of the ASA classifications produced by the computer were higher and two were lower than those produced by anaesthetists. The cost of a single evaluation by means of computer was significantly higher.

## Gynaecology

Jepson et al (1991) published a study which deals with the Apgar score. They concluded that the Apgar score is an important predictor of neonatal morbidity and mortality. However, in relation to long-term neurological effects, the Apgar score does not appear to offer a reliable prediction.

## Urology

Windsor et al (1996) studied the influence of the anaesthetic procedure and a risk score on the occurrence of silent cardiac ischaemia in the post-operative phase in 94 patients undergoing a transurethral prostate section (TUR). The choice of the anaesthetic procedure (spinal anaesthesia $N=60$, general anaesthesia $N=34$) had no influence on the incident of cardiac ischaemia. Existing symptoms of cardiac ischaemia and a high Detsky score had a higher risk of ischaemic events. Cullen et al (1994) studied the influence of age and ASA classification on morbidity and mortality in 1090 patients undergoing a TUR, a total endoprosthesis (TEP) or a cholecystectomy. The authors found that age and the ASA rating correlated with the duration of hospitalization and the occurrence of complications.

## Cardiothoracic–vascular surgery

Prause et al (1997a) compared two scoring systems with regard to the predictability of peri-operative mortality in thoracic surgery. The rate of peri-operative mortality in 845 patients was examined in the light of ranking in the ASA score and/or Goldman's CRI. Twenty-five patients died within the first 4 weeks after the operation. The ASA score demonstrated an independent correlation with the peri-operative mortality. However, a similar correlation could not be observed with Goldman's CRI. Koch et al (1996) studied the risk of peri-operative complications in coronary bypass surgery in women with the help of a new scoring system. Altogether 2800 patients (650 women) were investigated. The so-called illness scoring system includes 13 parameters. The results show that female sex alone is not a risk factor for an increase in morbidity or mortality in coronary bypass surgery. Higgins et al (1992) dealt with the same question. In a retrospective examination, they analysed 5051 patients undergoing a coronary bypass operation. A clinical scoring system which recorded various risk factors (emergency procedure, pre-operative serum creatinine levels greater than 168 μmol/l, severe left ventricular dysfunction, pre-operative haematocrit of 0.34, increasing age, chronic pulmonary disease, prior vascular surgery, reoperation and mitral valve insufficiency) in the peri-operative phase was used. This system also provides a prediction of morbidity and mortality. Weightman et al (1997) compared the prediction of risk of morbidity and mortality by four risk scoring systems in coronary bypass surgery. Four scoring systems which had been specially developed in Australia were used on 927 patients undergoing this operation. All of the scoring systems studied allowed a prediction of the peri-operative risk. None of them showed specificity or sensitivity. Hoffmann et al (1992) made a study using pre-operatively famed variables of the occurrence of peri-operative incidents and the long-term outcome in 653 patients undergoing heart valve replacement surgery. A correlation between pre-operative values and the risk of peri-operative complications and long-term outcome was also demonstrated. Piffare (1993) examined various risk factors in geriatric patients undergoing open-heart surgery. One hundred patients older than 75 years were assessed. Early mortality was at 3% and the rate of mortality after 2 years was at 25%. It was also possible here to distinguish pre-operative risk factors which allowed a prediction of mortality and morbidity. Chertow et al (1997) studied the risk of post-operative kidney failure in 43 642 patients undergoing cardiac surgery. The total risk of acute kidney failure was 1.1%. The 30 day mortality of these renal failure patients amounted to 63.72% and only 4.3% overall mortality. The risk of post-operative kidney failure can be relatively accurately assessed by means of data collected pre-operatively.

## Paediatric surgery

Hecker et al (1995) examined a risk score for the incidence of post-operative complications in paediatric surgery: 1425 operations on children were recorded and pre-operative risk scoring was carried out. The risk classification correlated well with the incidence of post-operative complication. Barbone et al (1993) examined complications in outpatient infant surgery. Because of the low complication rates in patients with ASA 1 and 2, there are no reasons to oppose outpatient infant surgery.

### Orthopaedic surgery

Arvidsson et al (1996) studied the prediction of post-operative incidents by means of four classification systems. A total of 1361 patients were assessed pre-operatively using this system which included the ASA rating, age, severity of the surgical intervention and a visual analogue scale for an intuitive assessment of risk. This system also offered a correlation between risk assessment and the incidence of post-operative complications.

## VALUATION

The prognosis or exclusion of peri-operative complications for the individual patient is not possible because statistical methods are not specific enough and the variance in individual values is too great. The causes of the complications are stated in the medical intervention. Recognizable or non-recognizable circumstances can appear which increase the difficulty of treatment and/or increase the risk as well as those which occur during the treatment, with appropriate care predictable and avoidable or not avoidable events. Incidents are complications that occur suddenly or unexpectedly and, because of possible grave consequences, a quick reaction of the attending doctor is necessary. Thereafter complications in anaesthesia are difficulties which occur pre-, intra- and post-operatively in the field of pain relief, preparation and accompanying measures as well as monitoring, maintenance and rehabilitation of the vital functions in comparison with the ideal typical process. The significance of the pre-operative estimation of the health state and of the operative risk lies on the one hand in the restriction of the surgical operation and in better peri-operative care with a better prediction of risk and on the other hand in the evaluation and comparison of similar groups. The routine use of a checklist can have practical consequences with regard to the planning and preparation of anaesthesia and surgery. An absolutely reliable prognosis of the anaesthetic risk is not possible but, because of the exact pre-operative description of the patient's state, the calculation of the risk becomes more reliable.

The ASA physical status classification has proven itself, because of its simplicity, rapid transparency and good corresponding judgement and classification of the situation of illness or health of surgical patients and for analysing the statistical risk worldwide.

The multifactorial CRI, the Mannheimer checklist and the Munich checklist have the advantage of higher accuracy and also a proven possibility of statistical risk prognosis, even though their use has not spread so far. Patient safety has been increased through exact judgement of age, cardiac status, necessity of operation, length of anaesthesia and surgery and laboratory results for more precise awareness and categorization of the anaesthetic risk and pre- and intraoperative interventions and monitoring measurements.

The assessment of the literature shows that the cardiac condition and cardiac events in the patient history, vessel diseases connected with changes in systemic blood circulation, and diseases of the lung connected with changes in the pulmonary function are the main risk factors for adverse outcomes in anaesthesia. Furthermore, diseases of metabolism connected with changes in laboratory values, history of smoking and age are important predictors for different outcomes in modern anaesthesia.

## REFERENCES


Arvidsson S, Quchterlony J et al (1996) Predicting postoperative adverse events. Clinical efficiency of four general classification systems. The project perioperative risk. *Acta Anaesthesiologica Scandinavica* **40(7):** 783–791.

*Barbone G, Montinaro L & Fiore T (1993) Ambulatory pediatric anasthesia. Personal experience. *Minerva Anestesiologica* **59(10):** 499–504.

*Browner WS, Du Chene Ag, Hulley SB et al (1992) Effects of the multiple risk factor intervention trial smoking cessation program on pulmonary function. A randomized controlled trial. *Western Journal of Medicine* **157(5):** 534–538.

Cassidy J, Marley A et al (1996) Preoperative assessment of the ambulatory patient. *Journal of Perianesthetic Nursing* **11(5):** 334–343.

Chijiiwa K, Yamaguchi K & Yamashita H (1996) ASA physical status and age are not factors predicting morbidity, mortality, and survival after pancreatoduodenectomy. *American Surgeon* **62(9):** 701–705.

Davies JM (1994) Comparison of selection of preoperative laboratory tests: the computer vs the anaesthesist. *Candian Journal of Anaesthesia* **41(12):** 1158–1160.

Detsky AS et al (1986) Cardiac assessment for patients undergoing noncardiac surgery. A multifactorial clinical risk index. *Archives of Internal Medicine* **146:** 2131–2134.

Forrest JB (1992) Multicenter study of general anaesthesia. III. Predictors of severe perioperative adverse outcomes. *Anesthesiology* **76(1):** 3–15.

*Goldman L, Caldera DL, Nussbaum SE et al (1977) Multifactorial index of cardiac risk in non cardiac surgical procedures. *New England Journal of Medicine* 7801.

*Goldman L, Caldera DL, Southwick FS et al (1978) Cardiac risk factors and complications in noncardiac surgery. *Medicine*, 7810.

Griffith KE, Tarala RA, Hall JL & Mander J (1994) Preoperative assessment and preparation. *International Anaesthesiology Clinics* **32(3):** 17–36.

Hall JL et al (1991) A multivariate analysis of the risk of pulmonary complications after laparotomy. *Chest* **99(4):** 923–927.

Hall JC, Ring-Mrozik E, Limmer S & Mantel K (1996) ASA status and age predict adverse events after abdominal surgery. *Journal of Quality Clinical Practice.* **16(2):** 103–108.

Hecker WC et al (1995) Risk score and postoperative complications in pediatric surgery. *Langenbecks Archiv für Chirurgie* **380(4):** 239–246.

Heino A, Mendeloff EN, Lilley RE et al (1992) Results of 500 general surgery patients operated on in the ambulatory surgery unit. *Annals of Chirurgic Gynaecology.* **81(3):** 295–299.

*Hennein HA, Estafanous FG, Loop FD et al (1994) Predictors of postoperative outcome after general surgical procedures in patients with congenital heart disease. *Journal of Peadiatric Surgery* **29(7):** 1994; 8666–8670.

Higgins TL, Vogt S & Roth J (1992) Stratification of morbidity and mortality outcome by preoperative risk factors in coronary artery bypass patients. A clinical severity score. *Journal of the American Medical Association* **268(14):** 1860.

Hoffmann A, Hemming AE, Allmann KG et al (1992) Heart valve substitution: the effects of preoperative findings on long-term outcome. *Schweizerische Medizinische Wochenschrift* **122(50):** 1907–1910.

Howell SJ et al (1997) Predictors of postoperative myocardial ischaemia. The role of intercurrent arterial hypertension and other cardiovascular risk factors. *Anaesthesia* **52(2):** 107–111.

Jepson HA, Talashek ML, Tichy AM et al (1991) The Apgar score: evolution, limitations, and scoring guidelines. *Birt* **18(2):** 83–92.

Koch CG, Higgins TL, Capdeville M et al (1996) The risk of coronary artery surgery in women: a matched comparison using preoperative severity of illness scoring. *Journal of Cardiothoracic and Vascular Anesthesia* **10(7):** 839–843.

Kvalsvik O, Fourtanier G, Fingerhüt A et al (1996) Selection of patients for ambulatory surgery. *Tidsskrift for den Norske Laegeforening* **116(4):** 500–503.

Lutz H (1972) The risk of general anaesthesia for surgical operations. *Deutsche Medizinische Wochenschrift* **24:** 7303.

Mangano DT, Browner WS, Hollentery M et al (1992) Long term cardiac prognosis following non-cardiac surgery. The Study of Perioperative Ischemia Research Group. *Journal of the American Medical Association* **268(2):** 233–239 (see comments).

Martin E (1992) Elderly patients—perioperative management from the viewpoint of the anaesthesist. *Fortschritte der Medizin* **110(13):** 235–237.

Masutani M (1992) Holter electrocardiographic findings in surgical patients during the perioperative period. *Masui* **41(3):** 401–412.

Menke H, Coetzee AR et al (1993) Predictive value of ASA classification of the assessment of the perioperative risk. *International Surgery* **78(3):** 266–270.

Van der Merwe WL, Uezono S, Nakata Y et al (1992) Pre-operative assessment and management of the patient with ischaemic coronary artery disease in non-cardiac surgery. *South African Journal of Surgery* **30(3):** 99–103.

O'Kelly B, Browner WS, Massie B et al (1992) Ventricular arrhythmias in patients undergoing non-cardiac surgery. The Study of Perioperative Ischemia Research Group. *Journal of the American Medical Association* **268(2):** 252–253 (see comments).

Owen WD et al (1978) ASA physical status classification. *Anaesthesiology* **49:** 239–243.

*Peter K et al (1980) Das Anaesthesierisiko. *Anästhesiologie Intensivmedizin Praxis* **9:** 240.

Pifarre R (1993) Open heart operations in the elderly: changing risk parameters. *Annals of Thoracic Surgery* **56 (supplement):** 71–73.

*Prause G, Offner G, Vicenti M et al (1997a) Comparison of two preoperative indices to predict peri-operative mortality in non-cardiac thoracic surgery. *European Journal of Cardiothoracic Surgery* **11(4):** 670–675.

*Prause G, Offner G, Vicenti M et al (1997b) Can ASA grade or Goldman's cardiac risk index predict peri-operative mortality? A study of 16,227 patients. *Anaesthesia* **52(3):** 203–206.

Tikkanen J, Hori-Viander M et al (1995) Death associated with anaesthesia and surgery in Finland in 1986 compared to 1975. *Acta Anaesthesiologica Scandinavica* **39(2):** 262–267.

Warner MA, Shields SE, Chute CG et al (1993) Major morbidity and mortality within 1 month of ambulatory surgery and anesthesia. *Journal of the American Medical Association* **270(12):** 1437–1441.

Weightman WM, Gibbs NM, Sheminant MR et al (1997) Risk prediction in coronary artery surgery: a comparison of four risk scores. *Medical Journal of Australia* **166(8):** 397–398 (see comments).

Windsor A, French GW, Sear JW et al (1996) Silent myocardial ischaemia in patients undergoing transurethral prostatectomy. A study to evaluate risk scoring and anaesthetic technique with outcome. *Anaesthesia* **51(8):** 728–732.

# 11

# Pre-operative anxiety, stress and pre-medication

WOLFGANG KRÖLL MD, PhD

Associate Professor

SUSANNE E. GASSMAYR MD

Resident

*Department of Anaesthesiology and Intensive Care Medicine, Karl-Franzens-University Graz, Auenbruggerplatz 29, A-8036 Graz, Austria*

The preoperative period means for the majority of patients a distressing situation, which is characterized by anxiety and fear. This is not only uncomfortable for the patient, but the simultaneously occurring activation of the sympathetic nervous system is potentially dangerous for a predisposed patient. Therefore, the primary goal for the patients preoperatively is to reduce anxiety and to induce sedation. Furthermore, if indicated, premedication should minimize the risk of an aspiration syndrome, prevent postoperative nausea and vomiting (PONV), provide analgesia, reduce secretions and control infections.

Besides fear and anxiety, stress may even cause an adaptation syndrome or depression. Physiological reactions of all organ systems to epinephrine and norepinephrine result from the stimulation of the sympathetic nervous system. To quantify these effects physiological and biochemical parameters are used. Fears may be recognized consciously or may be masked; for anxiety there is a differentiation between trait-anxiety and state-anxiety, which are of differing importance. It can be stated that the perioperative anxiety influences the patient's outcome.

For the preoperative medication both the individual patient, due to the physical and psychological status and to their history, and the desired goals have to be considered. The most commonly used ways of administration are oral, rectal or intranasal. We can choose our pharmaceutical premedication for anxiolysis and sedation from different substance classes as benzodiazepine, barbiturates, α-2-agonists, being aware of specific effects and side effects and also the possibility of antagonization. On the other hand, the anaesthesiologist has to know the meaning of the psychological premedication too.

Other unpleasant experiences for patients postoperatively are nausea and vomiting, which are to be treated prophylactically in patients with a known history of PONV. Anticholinergics are no longer routinely used for premedication, and from a legal point of view this is no longer recommended.

**Key words:** preoperative stress; premedication; PONV; anticholinergics.

*Baillière's Clinical Anaesthesiology*—
Vol. 12, No. 3, September 1998
ISBN 0–7020–2536–4
0950–3501/98/030485 + 11 $12.00/00

The practice of pharmaceutical pre-medication has changed and parallels the nowadays valid aims for pre-operative psychological preparation of patients; for decades the combination of an anti-cholinergic, analgesic and anti-histaminic drug has been administered i.m.; today benzodiazepines are given orally.

The primary goal for preparing patients before surgery is to reduce anxiety and to induce sedation; further considerations for pre-medication may be to minimize the risk of aspiration of gastric contents and to prevent post-operative nausea and vomiting (Lichtor and Zacny, 1994). Under special circumstances it can be necessary to provide analgesia, to reduce oral secretions and to control infections (Table 1).

**Table 1.** Aims of pre-operative preparation of the patient.

| |
|---|
| Anxiolysis: a decrease of the pre-operative level of anxiety combined with an emotional stabilization |
| Sedation: a decrease of the level of vigilance |
| Induction of sleep: an improvement of the sleep during the night before surgical intervention |
| Analgesia: relief of pain, if necessary, resulting in a decrease of the effects of pain-induced liberation of catecholamines |
| Vagolysis: inhibition of salivation and blockade of cardiovascular vagal reflexes |
| Prevention of post-operative nausea and vomiting (PONV) |
| Prophylaxis of aspiration |

## CAUSES OF PRE-OPERATIVE STRESS AND ANXIETY

During the peri-operative period the patient's situation is characterized by the influence of stressors, which can be defined as stimuli acting primarily on the brain and which secondarily induce reactions within the limbic system. When stress acts only briefly on the organism the characteristic emotions associated with it are fear and anxiety; for a longer duration the adaption syndrome will be the result (Tolksdorf, 1985).

Anxiety and fear are associated with an increase of the activity of the sympathetic nervous system leading to increased blood fluid concentrations of epinephrine and norepinephrine. The associated effects are an increase of the heart rate, cardiac output and blood pressure, an increased perfusion of brain and muscle, a dilation of the bronchi, a dilation of the pupils, a piloreaction and a decrease of the motility of the gut. Glycogen is mobilized, the blood glucose concentration increases and because of an increase of lipolysis the concentration of free fatty acids increases (Lichtor and Zacny, 1994; Tolksdorf, 1985).

The pre-operative increase of blood pressure and heart rate can lead to an increased myocardial oxygen demand; this will be dangerous for patients with decreased cardiac reserve and patients with pre-existing hypertension. A pre-operative hypokalaemia, induced by stress, may additionally lead to cardiac dysrhythmias.

The effects of stressors on the patient can be quantified by using physiological and biochemical parameters (Table 2). Out of these parameters only

**Table 2.** Quantification of pre-operative stress.

| Physiological parameters | Biochemical parameters | Metabolic parameters |
|---|---|---|
| Electroencephalogram | Cortisol | Blood glucose |
| Electrocardiogram | Adrenocorticotrophic hormone | Free fatty acids |
| Electro-oculogram | Prolactin | Potassium |
| Blood pressure | β-Endorphin | |
| Heart rate | Anti-diuretic hormone | |
| Capillary perfusion | Epinephrine | |
| Electrical activity of the skin | Norepinephrine | |
| Respiratory activity | | |

blood pressure and heart rate have gained popularity as routine parameters; as these are usually monitored during anaesthesia, clinically relevant changes from baseline are normally treated. From a practical point of view the interpretation of biochemical parameters is difficult and will not have any consequence for the daily routine.

The intensity of pre-operative anxiety differs interindividually and is correlated with a lot of various modifying factors (Götze, 1988; Badner et al, 1990).

- Fears recognized consciously by patients, which can even be expressed in a conversation between the patient, physician, nurse and relatives of the patient, include fears about the underlying disease, fears that the reason for surgery may be a malignant tumour, fears associated with anaesthesia, including fears of the needle stick, fears about intra-operative awareness and fears about feeling intra- or post-operative pain sensations as well as fears about post-operative changes in the familial, social or professional situation.
- Fears defined as 'masked' fears are not really recognized by the patient; they are displaced and can only be demasked during a talk between the patient and physician. This type of fear includes changes within the emotional area, such as increased irritability, increased nervousness, increase of anxiety or even a depressive feeling. Masked fears are further associated with changes in concentration and orientation, with development of psychovegetative reactions and finally with changes in the contact with the surroundings.
- Under special conditions, especially if the disease state is long lasting and is finally followed by a surgical intervention, the anxiety state of the patients can be complicated by various intensities of depression.

Two types of anxieties can be classified: trait anxiety as an attribute of the personality (dispositional anxiety) and state anxiety (situative anxiety) influenced by environmental events.

The level of pre-operative anxiety necessary to guarantee a good post-operative course is discussed controversially: results that demonstrate that a medium level of anxiety seems to guarantee a good outcome are in contrast to investigations which demonstrate that lower levels of pre-operative anxiety are correlated with a better outcome (Janis, 1958; Ramsay, 1972; Spielberger et al, 1973).

Trait anxiety does not change during the pre- and immediate post-operative period; state anxiety in contrast is dramatically increased 2 days before surgery and tends to decrease to acceptable values after the surgical intervention; the intensity of the decrease of the state anxiety is directly correlated with the individual level of trait anxiety. In contrast there are results showing that a positive correlation between the pre-operative level of trait and state anxieties exists; patients with a higher level of trait anxiety react with a higher intensity of state anxiety during the immediate pre- and post-operative period. In addition, the pre-operative level of trait and state anxieties also seems to be a predictor for the development of post-operative depressive disposition (Spielberger et al, 1973).

Neither the anaesthetist nor the nurse can accurately predict a patient's pre-operative anxiety level; the predictive accuracy, however, could be improved if the patients are specifically asked whether or not they are anxious.

In conclusion, the patient's personality and his or her coping style rather than concrete facts presented in a patient's medical history are responsible for the increased pre-operative stress load. This should continue in a reflexion about the usefulness of a standard pre-medication; moreover, an individual approach should be used in pre-operative medication (Egbert et al, 1963; Tolksdorf, 1984, 1985).

The degree of post-operative anxiety may influence the outcome of the patient; an increased and insufficiently treated stress load may result in an increased incidence of complications, a worsened reconvalescence with a longer-lasting stay in the hospital and worse results during the rehabilitation period. However, these considerations have not been confirmed. It could be shown that patients with sufficient information about surgery and anaesthesia show lower levels of state anxiety post-operatively, the need for analgesics was reduced and recovery quicker; other investigations, however, show that peri-operative anxiety and distress is not directly correlated with detailed information about surgery and anesthesia, but post-operative complications correlate well with the pre-operative level of information. In contrast, however, it can stated that information that is too detailed results in an increase of peri-operative anxiety. It has not been clarified why in some studies a significant effect was shown and in other investigations it could not be demonstrated; nevertheless, the reduction of pre-operative anxiety is a humane goal and should be attempted for each patient individually (Johnston and Vögele, 1993; Lichtor and Zacny, 1994; Roizen et al, 1996).

## PRE-OPERATIVE MEDICATION FOR ANXIOLYSIS, SEDATION AND ANALGESIA

To find the optimal drug or combination of drugs for pre-medication the individual goals have to be considered. In addition to anxiolysis the goals may be sedation, amnesia or if necessary analgesia. Furthermore, some patients require a decrease of autonomic responses, a prevention of PONV or a reduction of gastric volume and an increase of gastric pH; in other patients it could be reasonable to inhibit airway secretion, to take precautions against allergic reactions or to manage prophylaxis against infections. In a broad sense, continued therapy of concurrent disease has to be regarded as pre-medication (Duke and Rosenberg, 1996).

Principal factors for pre-medication are age and weight of the patient and the individual physical and psychological status including anxiety and reactions to pain; just as important as the physical examination is the history of the patient due to previous or actual diseases, allergies, previous PONV and drug use or abuse. There is a difference between our treatment of inpatients or outpatients and also the kind of planned surgical procedure influences the decision for pre-operative medication (Duke and Rosenberg, 1996).

In general pre-medication is administered orally for the patient's comfort and because of practicability on the ward; in paediatric anaesthesia rectal or intranasal application is prefered. In rare cases the pre-operative medication is administered intravenously, especially if a fast effect is desired, whereas the possibility of a transdermal medication of some substances or patient-controlled anxiolysis is probably of theoretical interest (Madler et al, 1996).

Substances used pre-operatively to achieve the different goals of pre-medication are listed in Table 3. Most commonly used for inducing anxiolysis are benzodiazepines, which bring further therapeutic effects such as anterograde amnesia, hypnosis and anti-convulsion. These effects are associated with minimal depression of ventilation and the cardio-

**Table 3.** Substances used pre-operatively.

| Classification | Drug | Dose*, route |
|---|---|---|
| Benzodiazepine | **Short acting** | |
| | Midazolam | 0.5–2 mg i.v. |
| | | 0.05–0.1 mg/kg i.m. |
| | | 0.5–1.0 mg p.o. |
| | | 0.2–0.3 mg/kg nasally |
| | Triazolam | 0.125–0.25 mg p.o. |
| | **Medium–long acting** | |
| | Flunitrazepam | 1.5–2.0 mg p.o. |
| | **Long acting** | |
| | Diazepam | 5–20 mg p.o. |
| | Dikaliumclorazepat | 40 mg p.o. |
| Barbiturates | Methohexital | 25 mg/kg rectally |
| | Secobarbital | 50–150 mg i.m., p.o. |
| | Pentobarbital | 50–150 mg i.m., p.o. |
| Ketamine | Ketamine | 2 mg/kg i.m. |
| | | 3 mg/kg nasally |
| | | 6 mg/kg p.o., rectally |
| $\alpha_2$-Agonists | Clonidine | 5 μg/kg p.o. |
| | Dexmedetomidine | 0.6 μg/kg i.v. |
| Opioids | Fentanyl | 15–20 μg/kg p.o. |
| | Sufentanil | 1.5–3.0 μg/kg nasally |

* Typical adult dose if not per kilogram.

vascular system. The advantage of this substance group is the possibility of their specific anatagonism of the central nervous system actions with flumazenil 8–15 mg/kg i.v. or antagonism of the sedation with aminophylline 1 mg/kg i.v.

The site of action of benzodiazepines is the α subunit of the γ-aminobutyric acid (GABA) receptor where they facilitate the binding of the inhibitory neurotransmitter GABA. This is followed by a flow of chloride ions into the cell, a hyperpolarization of the cell membrane and a resistance to excitation. The benzodiazepine receptor is almost solely found in the central nervous system which explains the minimal circulatory effects of benzodiazepines.

Midazolam is rapidly absorbed from the gastrointestinal tract, undergoes a first-pass hepatic effect (about 50%) and has a high degree of protein binding. It is two to three times as potent as diazepam; the injectable form is water soluble. The elimination half-life of midazolam is short (1–4 hours), increased in elderly and obese patients. Midazolam is mainly hydroxylated by microsomal liver enzymes and excreted in the urine as glucuronide conjugates. Newborns, especially immature and critically ill newborns, also metabolize midazolam slowly. For pre-medication remarkable interindividual differences have to be considered.

Diazepam has a fast gastrointestinal absorption, which leads to peak concentration in adults after about 1 hour and in children after 15–30 minutes. The intravenous solution contains propylene glycol and may cause pain and thrombophlebitis. Volume of distribution and protein binding are as high as for midazolam, but the elimination half-life is between 21 and 37 hours and even more prolonged in elderly patients. Diazepam is also metabolized by hepatic microsomal enzymes, and one principal metabolite (desmethyldiazepam) is nearly as potent as diazepam and may contribute to sustained or recurrent effects. The ultimate metabolites, mainly oxidized or glucuronide conjugated, are excreted in the urine.

Barbiturates are believed to produce their therapeutic effects also by acting on the GABA receptor complex (Christensen et al, 1994). They are metabolized by the liver (barbital and phenobarbital only to a small extent) and excreted by the kidney (Forth et al, 1987). An increase of hepatic microsomal enzyme will probably be seen after chronic use of barbiturates. Adequate sedation is reached with the disadvantage of a slight ventilatory and circulatory depression. Barbiturates are characterized by a long half-life time (4 hours–4 days) and are contraindicated in patients with porphyria (Stoelting and Miller, 1994).

Also effective for pre-medication are centrally acting $\alpha_2$-agonists stimulating inhibitory neurones in the medullary vasomotor centre (Stoelting and Miller, 1994). This results in a reduced outflow of sympathetic impulses to the periphery and a haemodynamic stability because of a decreased release of catecholamines by pre-operative anxiety and a blunted vegetative response to intubation and surgical stimulation. Centrally acting $\alpha_2$-agonists are sedative, anxiolytic and analgesic (presumably by activating the $\alpha_2$-receptors in the substantia gelatinosa), reducing the need for anaesthetics, diminishing the incidence of post-operative shivering, preventing muscle rigidity caused by opioids and decreasing the intraocular pressure; they are also anti-sialogenous and anti-emetic. Disadvantages are hypotension, bradycardia and dryness of the mouth and an obstructive hypoxaemia has also been described. The oral dosage of clonidine is 5 mg/kg body weight 90 minutes prior to induction. The pharmacokinetics of clonidine is characterized by good absorption after oral administration, excretion of about 60% unchanged in urine and an elimination half-life of 8.5 hours. A new highly selective and more potent $\alpha_2$-agonist is dexmedetomidine with a shorter duration of action. Dosages used are 2.5 mg/kg i.m. 1 hour prior to operation or 0.6 mg/kg i.v. 10 minutes before induction of anaesthesia (Aantaa et al, 1991; Mikawa et al, 1993; Scheinin et al, 1993; Nishina et al, 1995).

Pre-emptive analgesia is discussed controversially (Dahl et al, 1992; Katz et al, 1992). For pain relief in the pre-operative period there are potent analgesic drugs, for example opioids acting on five different receptors ($\mu_1$, $\mu_2$, $\kappa$, $\sigma$, $\varepsilon$). They are known to depress the respiratory centres and to cause muscle rigidity, histamine release and gastrointestinal problems but have the advantage of no direct myocardial depression. Hypotension because of stress reduction and vascular dilatation occurs. The elimination of opioids depends on the redistribution in lipid stores and afterwards on the hepatic metabolism and renal excretion (Faust, 1994).

Another analgesic with a certain sedative component applied pre-operatively is ketamine. It causes depression of the medial thalamic nuclei and of spinal cord activity. Metabolism occurs in the liver and excretion by the kidneys. Ketamine stimulates the sympathetic nervous system, increases the cerebral blood flow and may produce an emergency delirium. Therefore a combination with benzodiazepines is recommended (Faust, 1994).

For all pre-medicants you have to consider side-effects and interactions with concomitant medication and anaesthetics. Precaution is in general required for the use of depressant medication in newborn infants, elderly patients, patients with reduced level of consciousness or intracranial pathology and patients with severe pulmonary diseases or hypovolaemia.

Non-pharmacological methods are also assigned for the relief of anxiety in the pre-operative period. It is still the anaesthesiologists pre-operative visit which is of great importance. As well as the judgement of the history and of the physical status of the patient it is the anaesthesiologist's duty to rate the patient's psychological condition and to respond adequately in an empathic conversation. This is already documented by the study of Egbert et al (1963) where he could demonstrate that the pre-operative visit by an anaesthesiologist was more effective in relieving anxiety than the administration of barbiturates.

Apart from pre-medication, pre-operative assurance is not restricted to only the anaesthesiologist; everyone attending the patient should feel responsible. It could be shown that detailed information given to the patient reduces pre-operative anxiety. This information can also be conveyed by booklets, tapes or videos.

## PREVENTION OF POST-OPERATIVE NAUSEA AND VOMITING

Apart from pain sensations, nausea and vomiting is one of the most unpleasant experiences for patients during the immediate post-operative period. The incidence of PONV is about 25% (Wachta and White, 1992).

PONV can interfere with a variety of subjective and objective factors and therefore may put the optimal result of the surgical intervention into question. Post-operative nausea and emesis may lead to a significant decrease of patient's subjective well-being and may aggravate anxiety and pain immediately after emergence from anaesthesia. Furthermore, PONV can interfere with the surgical wound situation, as severe abdominal contractions can induce bleeding and haematoma formation in the surgical field. Aggravated emesis is associated with additional imbalances of the water and electrolye homeostasis (especially in patients at risk such as paediatric and geriatric patients). Post-operative mobilization of the patient is delayed owing to intractable emesis and immediately after emergence from anaesthesia PONV can lead to aspiration, especially when reflexes are not yet present (Clarke, 1984; Kröll, 1997).

The aetiology of PONV is multifactorial (Purkis, 1964; Dundee et al, 1965; Palazzo and Strunin, 1984; Kröll, 1997). A number of risk factors are responsible: patient-associated risk factors, surgery-associated risk factors, anaesthesia-relevant factors and post-operative risk factors (Table 4).

Patients with a previous history of PONV or a history of motion sickness show a three times higher incidence of emesis following anaesthesia and surgery; in female patients the incidence is two to four times higher than in male patients. Anaesthesia in younger people is associated with a twice higher incidence of PONV than in adults; in elderly people, however, the incidence of PONV seems to be decreased. Obesity, too short a period and a prolonged period of pre-operative fasting are also associated with an increasing incidence of nausea and vomiting.

Intra-abdominal surgical interventions and laparoscopic surgery are associated with an incidence of post-operative emesis of about 50–70%. Tonsillectomy, adenoidectomy and strabismus surgery as well as emergency surgical interventions are also associated with a high incidence of PONV.

**Table 4.** Risk factors for post-operative nausea and vomiting.

| Patient-associated risk factors | Surgery-associated risk factors | Anaesthesia-related risk factors | Post-operative risk factors |
|---|---|---|---|
| History of PONV | Intra-abdominal surgery | Etomidate | Post-operative pain |
| Motion sickness | Laparascopic surgery | Methohexital | Brisk movement |
| Female patients | Ear–throat surgery | Opioids | Hypotension |
| Children | Strabismus | Nitrous oxide | Hypoxia |
| Elderly patients | Orthopaedic surgery | Volatile anaesthetics | Hypercarbia |
| Obese patients | Emergency surgery | Difficult intubation | Early fluid intake |
| Short pre-operative fasting | | Regional anaesthesia | Psychological situation |
| Too long pre-operative fasting | | Duration of surgery | |

Etomidate and methohexital may increase the incidence of nausea and vomiting; propofol, in contrast, seems to have an anti-emetogenic effect. Nitrous oxide and opioids will increase the frequency of emesis during the post-operative period. The incidence of nausea and vomiting with the application of volatile anaesthetics ranges from 27% to 50% and regional anaesthesia is associated with a frequency of PONV of about 4–15%; the responsible causes may be hypoxaemia and hypotension. Further anaesthesia-relevant factors are the duration of surgery; in particular, long-lasting surgical interventions show an incidence of emesis of 46% (Kröll, 1997).

Post-operative pain is the main trigger of PONV during this period. Brisk movement of the patient immediately during the recovery period as well as hypotensive periods, hypoxia and hypercarbia may induce nausea and vomiting. Too early post-operative intake of fluids and psychological factors may be further responsible for this adverse event.

The affinities of drugs used as anti-emetics are listed in Table 5. The recommended doses of anti-emetic drugs are shown in Table 6 (Kröll, 1997).

**Table 5.** Affinity of anti-emetic drugs to the receptors.

| | $D_2$-receptor | Cholinergic receptor | Histamine receptor | Serotonin receptor |
|---|---|---|---|---|
| Phenothiazine | ++++ | ++ | ++++ | –/+ |
| Butyrophenons | ++++ | – – – – – – | + | –/+ |
| Anti-histamines | ++ | ++ | +++ | – – – – |
| Anti-cholinergics | + | ++++ | + | – – – – |
| Metoclopramide | +++ | – – – – – | + | ++ |
| 5-$HT_3$ antagonists | – – – – – – | – – – – – – | – – – – – | ++++ |

**Table 6.** Drugs for prevention of post-operative nausea and vomiting.

| Drug | Dose | Side-effects |
|---|---|---|
| Chlorpromazine | Prophylaxis: 5–10 mg p.o.<br>Treatment: 20 mg i.v. | Extrapyramidal symptoms, agitation, mouth dryness, sleep disturbances |
| Metoclopramide | Prophylaxis: 10 mg p.o., i.v.<br>Treatment: 10 mg i.v. | Extrapyramidal symptoms, diarrhoea, increase of prolactin concentration |
| Droperidol | Prophylaxis: 5–10 mg i.m.<br>Treatment: 5–10 mg i.v. | Extrapyramidal symptoms, sedation, hypotension |
| Atropin | Prophylaxis: 0.5 mg i.v. | Tachycardia, mouth dryness, sedation, delirium (elderly patients) |
| Ondansetron | Prophylaxis: 4 mg i.v.<br>Treatment: 4 mg i.v. | Headache, obstipation, flush |

## ANTI-CHOLINERGIC DRUGS

Anti-cholinergic drugs such as atropine, scopolamine and glycopyrrolate have been widely used for pre-medication (Table 7). Because of the change from i.m. application to oral application of pre-medicant drugs the use of anti-cholinergics has decreased; today from a legal point of view the use of these drugs is not recommended any more (List and Kröll, 1989).

**Table 7.** Effects of anti-cholinergic drugs.

| | Atropine | Scopolamine | Glycopyrrolate |
|---|---|---|---|
| Tachycardia | +++ | + | ++ |
| Inhibition of salivation | + | +++ | ++ |
| Sedation | + | +++ | 0 |
| Intraocular pressure ↑ | + | ++ | + |
| Anti-emetic | 0/– | +++ | 0 |
| Pressure of lower oesophageal sphincter ↓ | ++ | +++ | ++ |
| Temperature ↑ | + | ++ | +/++ |

However, for the following indications the application of anticholinergic drugs is obligatory: prophylaxis and treatment of bradycardia due to vagal stimulation (up to 2 mg), inhibition of increased salivation and inhibition of undesired side-effects of neostigmine used for antagonization of non-depolarizing muscle relaxants.

For the above indications anti-cholinergics should be given i.v., for which the duration of the effect is about 30 minutes; on i.m. application the full effects occur after 30–45 minutes and last for about 2 hours. An i.m. application is preferable to an i.v. application when the drug is used for inhibition.

Contraindications for the application of anti-cholinergic drugs in premedication are hyperthyreosis, full stomach and tachycardia (in patients with mitral insufficency and aortic stenosis). They can induce a central anticholinergic syndrome, especially in paediatric and elderly patients.

## REFERENCES


Aantaa R, Kanto J & Scheinin M (1991) Intramuscular dexmedetomidine, a novel alpha2-adrenoceptor agonist, as premedication for minor gynecological surgery. *Acta Anaesthesiologica Scandinavica* **35:** 283–288.

*Badner NH, Nielson WR, Munk S et al (1990) Preoperative anxiety: detection and contributing factors. *Canadian Journal of Anaesthesia* **37:** 444–447.

Christensen LQ, Bonde J & Kampmann JP (1994) Drug interactions with intravenous and local anaesthetics. *Acta Anaesthesiologica Scandinavica* **38:** 15–29.

Clarke RSJ (1984) Nausea and vomiting. *British Journal of Anaesthesia* **56:** 19–27.

Dahl JB, Hansen BL, Hjortso NC et al (1992) Influence of timing on the effect of continuous extradural analgesia with bupivacaine and morphine after abdominal surgery. *British Journal of Anaesthesia* **69:** 4–8.

Duke J & Rosenberg G (1996) *Anesthesia Secrets*, pp 104–105. Toronto: Hanley & Belfus.

Dundee JW, Kirwan MK & Clarke RSJ (1965) Anaesthesia and premedication as factors in post-operative vomiting. *Acta Anaesthesiologica Scandinavica* **9:** 223–231.

*Egbert LD, Battit GE, Turndor L & Beeches HK (1963) The preoperative value of the preoperative visit by an anaesthesist. *Journal of the American Medical Association* **185:** 553–555.

Faust RJ (1994) *Anesthesiology Review*, pp 123–128. New York: Churchill Livingstone.

Forth W, Henschler D & Rummel W (1987) *Pharmakologie und Toxikologie*, pp 500–503. B.I. Wissenschaftsverlag.

Götze P (1988) Psychische Führung des Patienten vor Anästhesie und Operation. In Rügheimer E & Pasch T (eds) *Vorbereitung des Patienten zu Anästhesie und Operation*, pp 322–331. Berlin: Springer.

Janis IL (1958) *Psychological Stress*. New York: Wiley.

*Johnston M & Vögele K (1993) Benefits of psychological preparation for surgery: a meta analysis. *Annals of Behavioral Medicine* **15:** 245–256.
*Katz J, Kavanagh BP, Sandler AN et al (1992) Pre-emptive analgesia: clinical evidence of neuroplasty contribution to postoperative pain. *Anaesthesiologi* **77:** 439–446.
Kröll W (1997) Postoperative Übelkeit und Erbechen. In List WF & Osswald PM (eds) *Komplikationen in der Anästhesie*, pp 711–719. Berlin: Springer.
Lichtor JL & Zacny JP (1994) Psychological preparation and preoperative medication. In Miller RD (ed.) *Anaesthesia*, 4th edn, pp 1015–1043. New York: Churchill Livingstone.
*List WF & Kröll W (1989) Ist eine Prämedikation mit Atropin noch zeitgemäβ? *Fortschritte der Medizin* **3:** 70–74.
*Madler C, Schmitt T & Poloczek S (1996) Prämedikation. *Anästhesiologie, Intensivmedizin, Notfallmedizin, Schmerztherapie* **31:** 509–524.
Mikawa K, Maekawa N, Nishina K et al (1993) Efficacy of oral clonidine premedication in children. *Anesthesiology* **79:** 926–931.
Nishina K, Mikawa K, Maekawa N & Obara H (1995) Oral clonidine premedication blunts the heart rate response to intravenous atropine in awake children. *Anesthesiology* **82:** 1126–1130.
Palazzo MGA & Strunin L (1984) Anaesthesia and emesis: I: ctiology. *Canadian Anaesthetists' Society Journal* **31:** 178–187.
Purkis IE (1964) Factors that influence postoperative vomiting. *Canadian Anaesthetists' Society Journal* **11:** 335–353.
Ramsay MAE (1972) A survey of preoperative fear. *Anaesthesia* **27:** 396–402.
Roizen MF, Klock PA, Klofta J et al (1996) How much do they really want to know? Preoperative patient interviews and anaesthesiologist. *Anesthesia and Analgesia* **82:** 443–444.
Scheinin H, Jaakola ML, Sjövall S et al (1993) Intramuscular dexmedetomidine as premedication for general anaesthesia: a comparative multicenter study. *Anesthesiology* **78:** 1065–1075.
Spielberger CD, Auerbach SM & Wadworth AP (1973) Emotional reactions to surgery. *Journal of Consulting and Clinical Psychology* **40:** 33–38.
Stoelting RK & Miller RD (1994) *Basics of Anesthesia*, p 114. New York: Churchill Livingstone.
Stoelting RK Handbook of Pharmacology and Physiology in Aesthetic Practice. Lippincott-Raven.
Tolksdorf W (1984) Das präoperative psychische Befinden. *Fortschritte der Medizin* **102:** 342–345.
Tolksdorf W (1985) *Der präoperative Stress*. Berlin: Springer.
Wachta MF & White PF (1992) Postoperative nausea and vomiting. *Anesthesiology* **77:** 162–184.

12

# Pre-anaesthetic fasting and aspiration

WERNER F. LIST MD

Professor and Chairman

GERHARD PRAUSE MD

Associate Professor of Anaesthesiology and Intensive Care Medicine

*Department of Anaesthesiology and Intensive Care Medicine, University of Graz, Auenbruggerplatz 29, A-8035 Graz, Austria*

The incidence of pulmonary aspiration of gastric content according to prospective and retrospective studies lies between 1.4 and 4.7 aspirations per 10 000 operations. Mortality has decreased to 1/71 829 anaesthesias. Reasons for an increased incidence of aspiration are higher American Society of Anesthetists status, emergency surgery, pregnancy and intestinal obstruction. New guidelines for elective surgical patients include no solid food for 6–8 hours but clear fluids up to 2 hours before operation. Acid antagonists and gastrokinetics should be given to patients with increased risk.

**Key words:** pulmonary aspiration; acute respiratory distress syndrome; incidence; risk factors; gastric volume, pH; pre-operative fasting; antacids; guidelines.

Mendelson (1946) first published his pathophysiology of acid aspiration as a syndrome. The so-called Mendelson syndrome includes pulmonary aspiration of acid stomach content, and consequently develops aspiration pneumonitis and acute respiratory distress syndrome (ARDS). Therapy of this syndrome is non-specific and symptomatic. Because of the high mortality of the aspiration syndrome anaesthesiologists try to prevent or minimize this danger in elective patients with the order of fasting of solid food and fluids after midnight, at least 6 hours before induction of anaesthesia. As well as the reduction of gastric content, an increase of the pH of the gastric juice above 2.5 will also decrease the risk of aspiration. It has been known for some time that clear fluids under normal conditions have a gastric emptying time of 1–2 hours and only solid particles have an emptying time between 6 and 8 hours. From this knowledge the n.p.o. order of 6–8 hours before operation has been questioned.

*Baillière's Clinical Anaesthesiology—*
Vol. 12, No. 3, September 1998
ISBN 0–7020–2536–4
0950–3501/98/030497 + 05 $12.00/00

## REASONS FOR PERI-OPERATIVE ASPIRATION

The most important factors are increased American Society of Anesthesiologists (ASA) status and emergency operations. The risk factors are as follows:

- low levels of consciousness;
- full stomach, pregnancy;
- recent ingestion of solid food;
- increased intra-abdominal pressure;
- gastro-oesophageal dysfunction;
- anaesthetic induction (difficult airway, intubation);
- extubation;
- drugs and opioids.

Contrary to the hypothesis of a slow gastric emptying in obese people it has been shown that gastric emptying is increased (Wright et al, 1983). In diabetic patients a gastroparesis has been hypothesized to be the reason for a slower gastric emptying of solid particles (Stoelting, 1997). Without question the residual volume of gastric juice of more than 25–500 ml (>0.4 ml/kg) as well as a pH below 2.5 play an important role.

## INCIDENCE OF PERI-OPERATIVE ASPIRATION

A number of prospective and retrospective studies each of more than 200 000 operations between 1980 and 1990 have shown that the general incidence is 1.4–4.7 aspirations per 10 000 operations (Stoelting, 1997). The diagnosis of aspiration is given if bilious juice or solid particles are found in the tracheal tree and if previously non-existent infiltrations are seen in the post-operative X-ray. In a retrospective study (Warner et al, 1993) the clinical significance of pulmonary aspiration during the peri-operative phase was studied from computer protocols. The incidence of aspiration in emergency operations was 1:895 and in elective surgical patients 1:3886. The overall incidence in 215 488 anaesthesias was 1:3216. Sixty-four percent of the patients who aspirated did not develop any further symptoms or X-ray abnormalities within 2 hours after aspiration and only 20% needed mechanical ventilation for more than 6 hours. Three of a total of 67 patients with aspiration died of ARDS. The total mortality of aspiration in 215 000 surgical operations was therefore 1:71 829 anaesthesias (Warner et al, 1993).

The procedure to prevent aspiration is a crash induction with endangered patients, pharmacoprophylaxis of acidity, positioning, cricoid pressure and removal of the gastric tube after suction before induction of anaesthesia. Pharmacoprophylaxis of acidity is as follows:

1. antacids (ranitidine, cimetidine, omeprazol) more than 2 hours before operation;
2. acid antagonists (sodium citrate 20–30 ml) 0–2 hours pre-operatively;
3. gastrokinetics (metoclopramide etc.) for volume reduction.

Nevertheless, Warner et al (1993) found in their retrospective study pulmonary aspiration in the same percentage with or without pharmacoprophylaxis. The routine use of pharmocoprophylaxis is not useful, is expensive and does not increase security. The application of a cricoid pressure has also being questioned.

## PHYSIOLOGY OF GASTRIC SECRETION

In normal adult patients gastric juice is produced continuously at 50 ml/hour; saliva is swallowed at about 70 ml/hour. The amount of gastric volume depends primarily on the frequency of gastric emptying. The removal of clear fluids is fast (half-life c. 12 min) so that 95% of the swallowed fluid is emptied within 1 hour. Gastric emptying of fluid depends on gastric distension and from the stomach–duodenum pressure gradient. Solid particles have to be liquefied and emptying may take up to 12 hours. About 50% of the solid particles are removed from the stomach within 2 hours after intake and can stay for up to 6 hours; clear fluids are completely removed after 2 hours. A slowed gastric emptying time is seen after trauma, pain and certain medications, especially opioids and atropine. Maltby et al (1988) found that pre-medication doses of opioids and atropine have no influence on the volume of gastric juice and pH, compared with unpremedicated adults. From case reports of intensive care patients with polytrauma it is known that solid particles can stay in the stomach for many days despite normal function and can be a reason for aspiration.

## STUDIES ON PRE-ANAESTHETIC FASTING

Phillips et al (1993) studied an elective surgical group of 100 adult patients, half of them with clear fluids up to 2 hours before operation (mean 400 ml), the other half having undergone 6 hours of fasting; gastric content and pH were investigated. Neither gastric fluid of about 20 ml in both groups nor the gastric pH around 2.5 was significantly different. In a double-blind study 136 ASA I–II patients were randomized into three groups. Group I with 8–10 hours fasting was compared with a group with 800 ml sugar-containing (12.5%) fluid in the evening and 400 ml water up to 2 hours before operation and a third group with the same amount of sugar-free sweetened fluid (1200 ml) (Lagerkranser et al, 1997). Patients with the sugared fluid showed a significantly improved well-being and less thirst and hunger until the post-operative phase. The intragastric volume was not different in the three groups, and the gastric pH was above 2.5 in the group with the sugar-containing fluids, significantly above the others. In children similar investigations with similar success were done (Schreiner et al, 1990). The majority of children with or without fluid from 10 hours up to 2 hours had a gastric volume of slightly more than 0.4 ml/kg and a pH of more than 2.5. No post-operative aspiration pneumonia occurred but children felt better with an n.p.o. order up to 2 hours before operation.

It therefore seems to be certain that the anxiety about clear fluids pre-operatively up 2 hours before an operation in children and adults increasing gastric content is not justified. If more than 2 hours have passed after intake of clear fluid, the endogenous gastric fluid secretion and gastric emptying time play the important role. If no pathological factors are present, swallowed fluids lead to an increased gastric emptying.

## GUIDELINE FOR PRE-ANAESTHETIC FASTING IN ELECTIVE PATIENTS

The safety of patients and patient comfort have to play the most important role. A change of guidelines for pre-operative fluid intake must not increase the risk of anaesthesia. All studies until now have shown that a liberalization of pre-operative fluid intake will not increase regurgitation or lead to an increased gastric volume. The integrity of the lower oesophagus sphincter will not be changed with fluid intake. Clear fluids do not lead to an increased risk of pulmonary aspiration and do not lead to an increased gastric volume. On the other hand, it should not be forgotten that solid food intake on the day of operation is not indicated because the gastric emptying time may be more than 6–8 hours. Each change of the n.p.o. order must carefully be discussed in the total organization of the hospital operating institutions.

### Guideline for adults

1. No solid food should be given later than 8 hours before the operation but up to 500 ml of clear fluid may be given up to 2 hours before operations; fluid administration with oral medication even 1–2 hours before the operative procedure if not more than 150 ml water are given.
2. Acid antagonists and metoclopramide for patients with increased risk of aspiration may be given if more than 2 hours of pre-operative time is left.
3. Sodium citrate may be used with acid gastric content in acute operations, for example with pregnancy and Caesarean section, if antacids are not indicated (less than 1–2 hours before operation).

### **Guideline for children** (Phillips et al, 1994)

1. No solid food should be given less than 6 hours before the operation.
2. Clear, possibly sugared, fluid (apple juice) may be given up to 2 hours before operation.
3. Antacids can be used with pathological gastrointestinal problems.

## REFERENCES

Lagerkranser M, Nygren J, Almström C et al (1997) Oral intake of a carbohydrate rich beverage pre-operatively improves safety and well-being. *Anaesthesia* **87A:** 952.

Maltby JR, Koehli N & Shaffer EA (1988) Gastric fluid volume, pH and emptying elective patients. Influences of narcotic-atropine premedication, oral fluid and ranitidine. *Canadian Journal of Anaesthesia* **35:** 562–566.

*Mendelson CL (1946) The aspiration of stomach content into the lung during obstetric anesthesia. *American Journal of Obstetrics and Gynecology* **52:** 191–205.

Phillips S, Hutchinson S & Davidson T (1993) Preoperative drinking does not affect gastric content. *British Journal of Anaesthesia* **70:** 6–9.

Phillips S, Diaborn AK & Hatch DJ (1994) Preoperative fasting for pediatric anaesthesia. *British Journal of Anaesthesia* **73:** 529–536.

Schreiner MS, Triebwasser A & Keon TP (1990) Suggestion of liquids compared with preoperative fasting in children. *Anesthesiology* **72:** 593–597.

*Stoclting RK (1997) NPO and aspiration: new perspectives. *ASA Annual Refresher Courses* **111:** 1–7.

*Warner MA, Warner ME & Weber JC (1993) Clinical significance of pulmonary aspiration during the perioperative period. *Anesthesiology* **78:** 56–62.

Wright RA, Krinsky S, Fleeman C et al (1983) Gastric emptying and obesity. *Gastroenterology* **84:** 747–751.

13

# Pre-anaesthetic evaluation

GORDON L. GIBBY MD

Associate Professor of Anesthesiology and Medicine

NIKOLAUS GRAVENSTEIN MD

The Jerome H. Modell, MD, Professor and Chairman of Anesthesiology

*University of Florida College of Medicine, Department of Anesthesiology, PO Box 100254, Gainesville FL 32610-0254, USA*

Pre-anaesthetic evaluation serves the purposes of maximizing both anaesthetic safety and efficiency of healthcare delivery. With the advent of outpatient care, the pre-anaesthetic evaluation clinic has become common. In the emerging American model, computerized records speed the gathering of patient records and the assessment of patient condition. Physician entry of patient evaluation is moving from dictation to direct physician entry, which will accelerate as handwriting and voice recognition systems mature. Purchasers of such systems should consider the security of the system, including authentication, authorization, encryption and storage systems utilized.

**Key words:** pre-anaesthetic evaluation; clinic; electronic medical record.

The goal of pre-anaesthetic evaluation is to maximize the safety of anaesthetic and surgical care, while minimizing the delays in obtaining that care. This must be accomplished in a way that also ensures and optimizes the efficient usage of the medical resources required to provide that care. Pre-anaesthetic evaluation goals are different for emergency and elective patients. For the emergency patient, maximum safety may be obtained by a swift evaluation to determine the most important aspects. For the elective case, a more leisurely pace of evaluation may allow for the correction of even minor medical problems that affect safety and for the careful planning that will most efficiently use the medical resources. Judgement is required. There is a wide difference between the cost of time spent during the pre-anaesthetic evaluation (which may utilize the time of only a few staff and may involve few highly paid staff) and time spent correcting problems during the intraoperative event. The latter can become extremely cost-intensive, expending time from both surgeon and physician, as well as surgical assistants and nurses as well as the high overhead expense of

*Baillière's Clinical Anaesthesiology—*
Vol. 12, No. 3, September 1998
ISBN 0–7020–2536–4
0950–3501/98/030503 + 19 $12.00/00

operating room time. Properly accomplished, a pre-anaesthetic evaluation can significantly improve peri-operative patient care and even, as an additional benefit, improve the financial performance of a surgical hospital.

## CURRENT US PRACTICE

The importance of pre-anaesthetic evaluation is often misunderstood in the United States. This is not surprising, because its costs are not specifically reimbursed by either American insurance companies, or the federal programs of Medicare and Medicaid. Even the Health Care Finance Administration's new Evaluation and Management Guidelines do not affect pre-anaesthetic care, because anaesthesiologists are paid on the basis of intraoperative time and complexity, with no weight given to pre-anaesthetic evaluation effort (Federal Register, 1996). The pre-anaesthetic and post-anaesthetic evaluations are merely required, and sometimes as little as a statement that the patient is 'an acceptable candidate for anaesthesia' will suffice. There has not been a randomized blinded anaesthetic outcome study to test whether pre-anaesthetic evaluations are of benefit, and because of current ethical concerns such a study is not likely. The problem of pre-anaesthetic evaluation is that the safety of anaesthesia has been so improved that the majority of patients may do well, perhaps even in the absence of anaesthetic planning. Only a minority of patients benefit significantly from pre-anaesthetic evaluation. This tends to make the anaesthesiologist minimize the benefit of the planning. However, the possibilities for the unfortunate are serious and reinforce the need to evaluate the patients.

Given this situation, it is the authors' opinion that the average department of anaesthesiology conducts pre-anaesthetic evaluations primarily because of requirement and because of a vague feeling that some level of planning would be beneficial. It is inconvenient to have to cancel a case on the day of surgery and embarrassing when the problem could have been detected and perhaps also corrected earlier.

The current practice of pre-anaesthetic evaluation varies widely in the United States, and there are no studies documenting the distribution of practice modes. The standard set by the American Society of Anesthesiologists (Figure 1) allows wide latitude in which personnel gather and correlate the information required, while placing the final responsibility on the anesthesiologist (American Society of Anesthesiologists, 1987). In some settings, pre-surgical patients are routinely seen by the primary physician, or by an internist, and 'cleared' for surgery. Of course, the value of the clearance is variable, and an anaesthesiologist must add an additional evaluation, however slight. Historically this was done the evening before at the patient's bedside. With the majority of patients now being admitted to the hospital on the morning of operation, this is no longer possible. Now, the anaesthesiologist's evaluation is often done at the bedside in the pre-operative holding area, where the anaesthesiologist is quite rushed. Previous medical records may be missing. Little patient teaching about the peri-operative process is possible, and the lack of earlier communication

BASIC STANDARDS FOR PREANESTHESIA CARE
(Approved by House of Delegates on October 14, 1987)

These standards apply to all patients who receive anesthesia or monitored anesthesia care. Under unusual circumstances, e.g., extreme emergencies, these standards may be modified. When this is the case, the circumstances shall be documented in the patient's record.

Standard I: An anesthesiologist shall be responsible for determining the medical status of the patient, developing a plan of anesthesia care and acquainting the patient or the responsible adult with the proposed plan.

The development of an appropriate plan of anesthesia care is based upon

1. Reviewing the medical record.
2. Interviewing and examining the patient to:
    1. Discuss the medical history, previous anesthetic experiences and drug therapy
    2. Assess those aspects of the physical condition that might affect decisions regarding perioperative risk and management.
3. Obtaining and/or reviewing tests and consultations necessary to the conduct of anesthesia.
4. Determining the appropriate prescription of preoperative medications as necessary to the conduct of anesthesia.

The responsible anesthesiologist shall verify that the above has been properly performed and documented in the patient's record.

**Figure 1.** Basic standard for pre-anesthetic evaluation as stated by the American Society of Anesthesiologists (1987).

with the patient by a member of the anaesthesiology department will probably cause increased cancellations as a result, for example, of patients misunderstanding nothing by mouth (n.p.o.) orders.

One accommodation to this change in practice is that many departments in recent years have added 'preop clinics' which have staffing ranging from full-time nurses trained to gather information for pre-anaesthetic evaluation to as-available staffing by anaesthesiologists. The impact of such clinics will vary with their thoroughness.

## THE EMERGING AMERICAN MODEL

The 'Anesthesia Preoperative Evaluation Clinic' at Stanford University is a good example and description of several better ways to accomplish pre-anaesthetic evaluation (Fischer, 1996). The physical arrangement of the clinic affects throughput and patient satisfaction. If possible, laboratory specimen drawing, electrocardiographic testing, echocardiography and simple chest radiography should be co-located with the clinic. A comfortable waiting room with educational materials for patients as well as a play area with safe toys for toddlers should be provided. An adequate number of offices and examining rooms should be provided so that evaluation will not be impeded by delays in properly locating patients. Because the pre-operative evaluation clinic is almost inevitably at least in part a walk-in clinic, as opposed to a scheduled one, the number of examination rooms should anticipate peak, not average, utilization. Examining rooms should also be structured to allow patients in wheelchairs to navigate easily. For those clinics with computerized records systems, the desk and patient chairs should be positioned so that the examiner can see the computer while still facing the patient, to maintain rapport. Location near the operating room is useful as it makes additional consultations quick and easy. There should also be a lounge area and office for the staff.

Staffing and scheduling are interrelated. An adequate number of clerks and professionals should be included to avoid undue delays. Typical times required to see patients vary with their complexity, with professional interviews by physicians taking roughly 27 minutes on average (Jackson et al, 1994), but considerably longer for patients with incomplete medical records. Nurses cross-trained with operating room experience are excellent for pre-operative teaching of patients. Direct person-to-person communication such as this has been found very useful to allay patients' pre-operative anxiety (Elsass, 1990), although the wealth of literature on anxiolytic premedicants demonstrates it may not always be adequate. Clerical staff and waiting room receptionists should be motivated to move patients politely through the system.

The flow of the patient through an ideal system might be as follows. After being greeted by the receptionist, patient identification, registration and insurance information (of great importance to the anaesthesia department for later billing) should be gathered and/or verified. This should be entered into a computerized billing system, ideally automatically connecting to a medical record system. For optimal communication with busy operating rooms in handling 'same-day' surgery patients, a visually appealing computerized tracking system may advise all clinic clerks and physicians, as well as operating room mangers, of the exact current status of each patient (Schwab et al, 1996). A simple questionnaire can be used to allow the patient to indicate their major concerns and medical problems (Figure 2).

## Nursing input

The next steps in the process heavily involve nursing. In the United States, the Joint Commission on Accreditation of Healthcare Organizations (JCAHO), a unifying body that performs self-policing of hospitals and other healthcare institutions, requires that nursing departments of hospitals provide comprehensive peri-operative care and education. This must include pre-operative care and education. It is therefore quite natural for vital signs to be gathered and patient education as to the expected train of events to be provided by nurses cross-trained with operating room experience. Educational pamphlets and videotapes may assist with this practice.

Items that may best be accomplished by the nursing staff include

- checking that critical steps in the pre-operative path have been achieved,
- preparing the patient for the surgery psychosocially,

42351

College of Medicine at the University of Florida

**Patient Medical History**

Medical Record Number

BP Systolic — BP Diastolic — Weight (Pounds) — Diagnosis — Age(yrs) — Height-Ft — Inches — Month/Surg — Day/Surgery — Surgical Resident Beeper for questions regarding this patient

Patient Last Name

Patient First Name

TO THE PATIENT: Please BLACKEN IN (not make an X) the YES or NO circle for each of the following medical conditions, if you HAVE HAD, or CURRENTLY HAVE the condition.

**1**

| Yes | No | | Yes | No | | Yes | No | |
|---|---|---|---|---|---|---|---|---|
| ○ | ○ | 1. Loose teeth, or dentures | ○ | ○ | 14. Asthma (wheezing) | ○ | ○ | 28. Abnormal bleeding |
| ○ | ○ | 2. Seizures (convulsions) | ○ | ○ | 15. Pneumonia | ○ | ○ | 29. Sickle Cell disease |
| ○ | ○ | 3. Blackouts (syncope) | ○ | ○ | 16. Shortness of breath | ○ | ○ | 30. Weak Eye Movements |
| ○ | ○ | 4. Stroke | ○ | ○ | 17. Bronchitis/emphysema | ○ | ○ | 31. Pregnant now? |
| ○ | ○ | 5. Paralysis or handicap | ○ | ○ | 18. Smoking | ○ | ○ | 32. Back Trouble |
| ○ | ○ | 6. High Blood Pressure | ○ | ○ | 19. Cold in last 2 weeks | ○ | ○ | 33. High fever after anesth. |
| ○ | ○ | 7. Heart Attack (M.I.) | ○ | ○ | 20. Heartburn | ○ | ○ | 34. Family History of anesthesia problems |
| ○ | ○ | 8. Angina or Chest Pain | ○ | ○ | 21. Hiatal Hernia | ○ | ○ | 35. Thyroid Trouble |
| ○ | ○ | 9. Irregular heartbeat | ○ | ○ | 22. Hepatitis or Jaundice | ○ | ○ | 36. Alcohol beverages daily |
| ○ | ○ | 10. Palpitations | ○ | ○ | 23. Kidney Trouble | ○ | ○ | 37. Ulcers |
| ○ | ○ | 11. Heart Failure | ○ | ○ | 24. Diabetes | ○ | ○ | 38. Arthritis |
| ○ | ○ | 12. Must sleep upright or on several pillows to breathe | ○ | ○ | 25. Low Blood Sugar | ○ | ○ | 39. Will accept blood transf. |
| ○ | ○ | 13. Rheumatic fever | ○ | ○ | 26. Blood clotting problems | ○ | ○ | 40. Have autologous blood |
| | | | ○ | ○ | 27. Have cancer? | ○ | ○ | 41. Previous difficult airway |
| | | | | | | ○ | ○ | 42. Have you signed an Advance Directive? |
| | | | | | | ○ | ○ | 43. Other problems |

**2** Please enter the names of up to FOUR of your medications in block capital letters.
○ **Blacken here if more than 4**

**3** Please print here a telephone number where you can be reached the night before your surgery between 5 and 7 PM.
area code — phone number

**4** **Please list any medications to which you are allergic, and briefly note the reaction**
○ **Blacken if MORE THAN TWO Allergies to medications**

**THANK YOU** for completing this medical history. It will help our physicians better care for you.

Office Use Only
○ Bring into clinic ○ Doesn't have to come in ○ Phone call was reqd
Reviewing Physician — Signature(s)

Preop Pt Hx #5 ID on IV 425Ln V1.05 4/27/95 Copyright 1995 Gordon L Gibby MD

**Figure 2.** Basic medical history tool used at the University of Florida for pre-anaesthetic patients. This form can be scanned electronically into a database if desired.

- educating the patient about procedures for arrival and admission to the hospital and
- gaining an understanding of the normal daily routine of the patient.

To ensure that the process may efficiently continue, the nurse may verify that the previous steps have been properly completed, including

1. history and physical (H&P) and vital signs recorded on chart
2. old chart available if extant
3. hospital card available
4. proper operative permit

5. minimum pre-operative laboratories appropriately ordered by protocol (if any)
6. availability of autologous or directed donor blood

Information that may be gathered by the nurse includes

1. documentation of allergies (including latex) and their reactions
2. documentation of current medications
3. assessment and documentation of language and method of reaching family members
4. assessment of anxiety level and coping skills
5. documentation of skin condition and integrity

Education that may be accomplished by the nurse includes the following:

1. explanation of 'advance directives' to allow documentation of the patient's wishes in the event of a terminal health problem and imminent end of life;
2. discussion of pre-operative holding, operating room, post anaesthesia care unit (PACU) routines, and locations where family members may wait during surgery;
3. discussion of post-operative pain management, early ambulation, pneumatic compression devices, dressing, tubes and drains, and pre- and post-operative routines for ward and intensive care unit;
4. review of important instructions, emphasizing n.p.o. orders, requirements for outpatients to have someone to take them home, and arrival instructions, including determining the arrival time required.

## Anaesthesia evaluation

On the basis of the results of the patient questionnaire (or previous review of the referring surgeon's history and physical), patients with more straightforward problems may be seen by registered nurse practitioners (RNPs). The more complicated patients may be seen by physicians or with advice given to the RNP from an attending or resident.

There are multiple important areas of evaluation which should be completed by the physician or specially trained nurse practitioner to allow the proper decision making to occur for the anaesthetic. These include the following:

1. accurate and unique identification of the patient;
2. careful description of the surgical diagnosis and procedure planned;
3. name of the surgeon;
4. known types of anaesthesia requested by the surgeon, if any;
5. date of the planned operation;
6. history of the present surgical illness;
7. review of the patient's body systems, to include the central and peripheral nervous system, cardiovascular system, pulmonary systems, gastrointestinal system, haematological, endocrine, skeletal, integumentary and psychosocial systems;

8. allergies and the allergic response, including those to latex;
9. habits of abuse of tobacco, alcohol and any illicit drugs;
10. medications, both prescription and over the counter (non-prescription);
11. vital signs, including height, weight, blood pressure (site noted), pulse rate and quality, respiratory rate and, often, room air pulse oximetry;
12. physical examination at a minimum to include general appearance and habitus, airway, respiration, cardiovascular evaluation;
13. laboratory results ordered and obtained previously by the surgeon, or any indicated laboratory results deemed necessary by the anaesthesiologist;
14. past surgical and associated anaesthetic history and family history of anaesthetic problems.

In previous years, various protocols have been used for screening laboratory testing (Roizen, 1994). With looming financial insolvency, the US Federal Medicare and Medicaid programmes (both administered by Health Care Financing Administration (HCFA)) decided in 1996 to require a sign, symptom or diagnosis (rather than just 'pre-operative laboratory test') before any laboratory test cost can be reimbursed (Painter, 1997). HCFA has now refused to reimburse for blanket test 'batteries' and instead requires billing for individual tests within the previously common batteries (Auxter, 1998). This has ended the use of protocols in many locations, and the requirement to treat federally reimbursed patients identically to all others has meant that these changes have affected all patients. The American Society of Anesthesiologists has released a position that requires no basic screening tests (see Figure 3).

A substantial financial impetus for the establishment of pre-anaesthetic evaluation clinics, and also for the usage of electronic patient data gathering tools (Davies et al, 1994), has been the reduction in laboratory tests possible

STATEMENT ON ROUTINE PREOPERATIVE LABORATORY AND DIAGNOSTIC SCREENING
(Approved by House of Delegates on October 14, 1987 and last amended on October 13, 1993)

Preanesthetic laboratory and diagnostic testing is often essential; however, no routine* laboratory or diagnostic screening** test is necessary for the preanesthetic evaluation of patients. Appropriate indications for ordering tests include the identification of specific clinical indicators or risk factors (e.g., age, pre-existing disease, magnitude of the surgical procedure). Anesthesiologists, anesthesiology departments or health care facilities should develop appropriate guidelines for preanesthetic screening tests in selected populations after considering the probable contribution of each test to patient outcome. Individual anesthesiologists should order test(s) when, in their judgment, the results may influence decisions regarding risks and management of the anesthesia and surgery. Legal requirements for laboratory testing where they exist should be observed. The results of tests relevant to anesthetic management should be reviewed prior to initiation of the anesthetic. Relevant abnormalities should be noted and action taken, if appropriate.

* Routine refers to a policy of performing a test or tests without regard to clinical indications in an individual patient.
** Screening means efforts to detect disease in unselected populations of asymptomatic patients.

**Figure 3.** American Society of Anesthesiologists (1993) statement of pre-anaesthetic laboratory screening tests.

when surgeons and anaesthesiologists agree to allow the anaesthesiologist to choose the applicable laboratory tests. The costs savings associated with more appropriate utilization of pre-operative testing offset the costs associated with the operation of a pre-anaesthetic evaluation clinic. Now that an indication is required for any laboratory test, at least for federal payers in the United States, it is possible that these savings may become the norm.

After all the patient medical information is gathered and reviewed, the anaesthesiologist discusses the range of possibilities of anaesthetics for the planned procedure, leaving the actual intraoperative anaesthesiologist the maximum possible discretion in the final choice of anaesthesia. The choices considered acceptable to the patient should be documented, and informed consent obtained and documented for all consented options of anaesthesia, with witness of that consent by a third person on the hospital staff.

Much of the process of pre-anaesthetic evaluation is data gathering. In addition to the anaesthesiologist's review of systems, physical examination, review of past medical and surgical history, obtaining relevant items of pre-existing medical records for review is extremely important. At a minimum, this includes the surgical history and physical, which may reveal items missed by the anaesthesiologist, as well as previous pre-anaesthetic or intraoperative records from the institution. Other items of interest include previous radiographic or computed tomography or magnetic resonance imaging studies, previous electrocardiographic and echocardiographic studies, previous cardiac catheterization, stress electrocardiography, dobutamine stress echocardiography, thallium cardiac ischaemia evaluations and Holter monitor studies. Previous consultations from pulmonary, neurological, neurosurgical, cardiology and cardiothoracic departments will often be important. When these items exist, but are not available to the pre-anaesthetic evaluation clinic, it causes delay and makes necessary additional work to obtain them, and results in a considerably longer patient evaluation timespan. This substantially slows down the evaluation clinic throughput. One study demonstrated that 29% of patients were missing extant information, and that the patients missing external information required on average more than 30 minutes longer evaluation time than those not missing external information (Gibby et al, 1996b; Gibby and Schwab, 1998). The pre-anaesthetic clinic should work with surgeons and nurses to give the patient a clear understanding from the earliest contact that significant previous work-ups should be brought with the patient to the pre-anaesthetic clinic.

In practice in the United States, it is most common for a printed form to be used to guide the gathering of data for the anaesthesiologist. This has the advantage of increasing standardization within one institution, and reducing variability in the quality of the evaluation. However, across the nation, there has been little standardization of forms (Figures 4 and 5). Informed consent may be documented using a standard form or, even better, a specific consent for the planned anaesthetic. The major medical value is in the discussion with the patient to inform them truly of the risks and benefits of the anaesthetic options available.

Paper records cause a number of problems in the transfer of information to the pre-anaesthetic evaluation clinic and later to the anaesthesiologist.

UAB DEPARTMENT OF ANESTHESIOLOGY **PREANESTHETIC EVALUATION**

PROPOSED OPERATION | HT

PREOPERATIVE DIAGNOSIS | WT

| BP | HR | RR | TEMP | PHYSICAL STATUS 1 2 3 4 5 E |
|---|---|---|---|---|

**SYSTEMS REVIEW AND PAST MEDICAL HISTORY**

NEURO SEIZURE ___ TIA ___

ENT IMPAIRED HEARING ___ BLIND ___

CV HTN ___ ANGINA ___ $^{\circ}$/o MI ___ CHF ___ PALPITATIONS ___ MURMUR ___

EXERCISE TOLERANCE ___

RESP ASTHMA ___ BRONCHITIS ___ COUGH (PRODUCTIVE) ___ DYSPNEA ___

GI REFLUX ___ PUD ___ HEPATITIS ___

GU ESRD ___

GYN PREGNANT? ___ EXCESSIVE MENSES ___

ORTHO ARTHRITIS ___ LOCATION ___ MUSCULAR DZ ___

HEME BLEEDING DYSCRASIA ___ SICKLE CELL ___

ENDO DM ___ THYROID ___

COMMENTS: ___

**PAST SURGICAL HISTORY/PAST ANESTHETIC HISTORY** BLOOD TRANSFUSIONS ___

**FAMILY HISTORY/ANESTHETIC COMPLICATIONS**

**SOCIAL HISTORY**

Tobacco ___ ETOH ___ IVDA ___

**PHYSICAL EXAM**

NEURO ALERT ___ ORIENTED X ___ DEFICITS ___

AIRWAY

ORAL OPENING ADEQUATE ___ MARGINAL ___ POOR ___

DENTAL GOOD ___ POOR ___ DENTURES ___ CAPS ___

NECK ROM ADEQUATE ___ MARGINAL ___ POOR ___

CHEST CTA ___

CV RRR ___

OTHER ___

**ANESTHESIA PLAN/CONSENT**

R/B/I GETA ___ REGIONAL ___

MAC ___ DISCUSSED

INDICATES UNDERSTANDING ___ CONSENTS ___

MONITORS: A-LINE ___ CVP ___ PA CATH ___

FIBEROPTIC ___ JET VENTILATOR ___

**PRE-OP HOLDING ORDERS**

IV FLUIDS ___

PREFERRED SITE ___

SUGGESTED SIZE ___

MEDS ___

OTHER ___

RESIDENT/CRNA DATE ATTENDING ANESTHESIOLOGIST

25139 Rev. 2/91 MEDICAL RECORD

**CURRENT MEDICATIONS**

**ALLERGIES**

**LAB RESULTS**

Na ___ K ___ Cl ___ $CO_2$ ___

Glu ___ BUN ___ Cr ___

Hgb ___ Hct ___ Plt ___ WBC ___

PT/PTT

ABG's

EKG

CXR

OTHER

**HOLDING AREA NOTES**

NAME ID ___ CONSENT ___ NPO ___

H&P ON CHART ___ EKG ON CHART ___

IV FLUID ___

IV SIZE/SITE ___

PRE-OP MEDS GIVEN: PEPCID ___ REGLAN ___

VITAL SIGNS BP HR RR $SaO_2$

| TIME | DRUG | STENGTH | ROUTE |
|---|---|---|---|
| | | | |
| | | | |

NOTES ___

NURSE

**Figure 4.** Representative pre-anaesthetic evaluation form. From the Department of Anesthesiology, University of Alabama.

Paper records may be voluminous, leading to 'volumes' and possibilities of incomplete records. Shadow charts may be kept by clinics that do not participate in the institutional record. Illegibility is rife, and authorship of the record is sometimes questionable; changes may be hidden, data are unstructured and cannot be used by multiple physicians simultaneously. It is difficult and time consuming to obtain records from distant institutions. Because the business of the pre-anaesthetic clinic is critically dependent on gathering information, documenting it, drawing conclusions and documenting the conclusions, these deficiencies of the paper medical record are serious impediments.

| | LOCATION DATE SERVICE |
|---|---|
| UNIVERSITY OF MICHIGAN HOSPITALS | |
| ANESTHESIOLOGY PRE-OPERATIVE/POST-OPERATIVE EVALUATIONS | Reg. No. Class |
| PATIENT NOTES ☐ INPATIENT ☐ OUTPATIENT | Name |
| Date: ______ | Address |

ANESTHESIOLOGY PRE-OPERATIVE EVALUATION

H.P.I.:

PROCEDURE:

R.O.S.:

PAST ANESTHESIA Hx:

FAMILY Hx OF ANESTHESIA PROBLEMS:

ALLERGIES:

MEDICATIONS:

PHYSICAL EXAM: Naso-oral pharynx ______

Blood Pressure: ______ Lungs ______

Pulse: ______ Weight: ______ Heart ______

LABS:

☐ The risks of Anesthesia were discussed with the patient who understood and consented.

☐ ASA Risk Factor: ______

Anesthetic Technique:

☐ Pre-Medication Ordered ☐ Consent Signed

☐ The plan for Anesthetic Management was discussed with Dr. ______

SPECIAL CONSIDERATIONS:

STAFF ANESTHESIA NOTES:

Signature/Date: ______ (Flip up and over for Post-Operative Evaluation)

| H-2051104 Rev. 8/87 | THIS FORM MUST REMAIN IN MEDICAL RECORD | MH University of Michigan Medical Center | ANESTHESIOLOGY PRE-OPERATIVE/ POST-OPERATIVE EVALUATIONS |
|---|---|---|---|

**(INPATIENTS ONLY)**

ANESTHESIOLOGY POST-OPERATIVE EVALUATION

Date: ______ Time: ______

RECOVERY FROM ANESTHESIA:

HEMODYNAMIC STATUS:

RESPIRATORY STATUS:

OTHER:

ANESTHESIA RELATED COMPLICATIONS:

RECOMMENDATIONS:

Signature/Date: ______

**Figure 5.** Another pre-anaesthetic evaluation from. From the University of Michigan Hospitals.

## ELECTRONIC MEDICAL RECORDS IN THE PRE-ANAESTHETIC CLINIC

The continued development of electronic medical records should provide solutions for many of the problems described, as shown in Table 1. Within one's own institution, electronic medical records should be advocated whenever possible. For the pre-anaesthetic evaluation of patients, Tompkins et al (1980) demonstrated a computerized system capable of performing significant portions of the interview. There are now many electronic medical record systems available, from the interview systems such as the HealthQuiz (Lutner et al, 1991) to physician-operated systems integrated with intraoperative record keepers. These systems may be divided into types of systems by user-interface as follows:

- paper imaging systems that make it easy for later physicians to see the handwritten pre-anaesthetic evaluation;
- click yes–no systems with options for free text additional typing;
- click systems with problem-oriented canned text and ability for additional entry (Gibby et al, 1996c);
- voice recognition systems (Smith et al, 1990) (which have the disadvantage that the patient can hear your conversation if you do not leave the room);
- pen recognition systems, usually with additional clickable text.

The advantages of such systems over paper records are summarized in Table 1 (East, 1992).

The field of anaesthesiology should strive toward a database of structured characterizations of patients and their treatment with the resulting outcome. Such a system would allow for far more accurate and real-world analysis of risk–benefit of various types of treatment in differing patient populations (O'Rourke and Smith, 1975; Louagie et al, 1995; Gibby, 1997). Such systems would eventually allow better prediction of patient outcomes (Jackson et al, 1993). Such a system can only be achieved with the wide use of electronic medical records (McDonald and Tierney, 1988; Edsall, 1991) (pre-anaesthetic, intraoperative and post-operative) and with a method for 'scrubbing' the patient identity from these records and combination of standard extracts of these records into a large national database. The Society for Technology in Anesthesia in the United States has

**Table 1.** Advantages of electronic clinical information systems over paper records (East, 1992).

| Service | Method |
|---|---|
| Data sharing | Simultaneous access to data |
| Data consistency | Error checking, constraints |
| Data security | Authorization controls |
| Data protection | Back-up, recovery, transaction controls |
| Data timeliness | Immediate availability to all authorized users |
| Data standards | Data definitions for database entry |
| Data use | Queries, retrievals, reports |

expressed its support for such a development (Society for Technology in Anesthesia, 1998). The technology for the collection exists, but it is unclear how the individual patient identity removal would be accomplished. This is a necessary feature to preserve patient confidentiality. Such electronic anaesthesia information systems would also facilitate the development of easily accessible registries of patients with significant hidden risks or previous anaesthesia problems (Mark et al, 1996; Lack et al, 1994).

In choosing an electronic pre-anaesthetic evaluation system several aspects should be evaluated (Table 2). For the long-range benefit to the institution, it is important to obtain the system with the highest level of structured data entry and storage, while also maintaining the highest level of user ease; these are conflicting goals in many cases. Regardless of these ideal considerations, user satisfaction will have to be the highest priority, because in a setting where electronic medical records are novel, an unpopular system that is not used will have a severely adverse impact on the development of retrievable electronic medical records (Dambro et al, 1988). Physicians can be more demanding than other staff (O'Dell et al, 1991). Surprisingly, in at least one system, physicians were willing to enter substantially more information into a computer than they normally penned (Safran et al, 1991). Usage of e-mail at Yale University had reached 32 messages per person per month, suggesting that simple keyboard-based systems are finding acceptance (Grajek et al, 1997). Structured data entry and storage, however, are important: they allow for easy patient data retrieval by identification number, by name, type of case, date or any of several additional items. Without structured data entry and storage, administrative overview and practice review (extremely useful in the realm of managed care (American Society of Anesthesiologists, 1996) are virtually impossible (Wyatt, 1994), but the concept of structured data entry is quite different from typical paper records (Stead and Hammond, 1983; Stead et al, 1983). Structured data entry and storage also impose severe requirements on even current databases (Thompson et al, 1995).

**Table 2.** Important characteristics of electronic medical records.

| |
|---|
| Structure in data storage and retrieval |
| User input interface |
| Possibilities for electronic signatures |
| Type of operating system |
| Display technology and capabilities |
| Presentation technology |
| Screen layout characteristics |
| Data storage technology |
| Back-up technology |
| Network technology |
| Journalling methods |
| Security procedures |
| External communications protocols |
| Printing technology |
| Availability of immediate CPT and/or ICD-9 coding of cases |
| Ability to integrate information in a peri-operative patient flow |
| Training requirements |

Voice recognition systems are often requested by naive physicians, but one product discontinued the feature. Voice input may be even slower than handwriting recognition (Bergeron, 1996) and has the continuing disadvantage that the patient may overhear sensitive material.

A fully structured pre-anaesthetic medical record would allow immediate access to any medical problem by type and would have structured characterizations of the problem, such as onset, duration, severity, diagnostic and therapeutic efforts. Such detailed characterization of patient medical problems was found to be financially beneficial to the hospital in a study of prospective reimbursement (Gibby et al, 1997a). The mechanism of improved reimbursement was as follows. HCFA diagnosis-related group prospective reimbursement is designed to control federal health expenditures by paying fixed amounts for patients who fall into specific medical categories, causing the hospital to absorb the risk of variable actual hospital costs. These prospective reimbursements are greater for patients with co-morbid problems, but only if the co-morbid problem shifts the patient into a different diagnosis-related group. If the hospital fails to recognize that the patient fits into the more complicated category, the hospital will be erroneously underreimbursed (Hsia et al, 1992): 1.5% of patients were found to be justifiably upgraded in category based on information that coders found in the pre-anaesthetic structured evaluation, which was not seen elsewhere in the chart.

Paper imaging systems, while relatively easy to implement and require only scanning of the pre-anaesthetic evaluation, have extremely minimal structure and suffer from the inconsistent legibility of the physician or nurse recorder. They are, however, a reasonable minimum for a modern healthcare facility.

Click yes–no systems with the option for free text additional typing are designed to allow the minimal structured pre-anaesthetic evaluation to be most easily entered into the computerized system. However, such systems may discourage entry of additional characterization of the patient's problems and decrease their usefulness in transferring information to the caregiver. This is clear because, even in the creation of a simple physical examination, it required 131 clickable phrases to accommodate even 30% of evaluations in one study (Murphy and Barnett, 1996), suggesting that even canned-text systems will require significant additional typing, in agreement with the findings of Gibby et al (1996c), who found that only approximately 50% of the characters in the review of systems could be supplied by a substantial visual list of clickable text. It is best to make it easily possible to select structured text, while also allowing additional free text entry (Figure 6).

There have been very few evaluations of the impact of such direct physician-entry systems on the professional time involvement. Obviously the keyboard–mouse technology has the potential to slow significantly evaluation by those who are not competent typists (Tierney et al, 1993) but still preserves the ability to gather older information and to obviate the need for re-entry, even by a pencil. Jackson et al (1994) found that one keyboard–mouse system had no impact on the physician time involvement in a resident-teaching hospital.

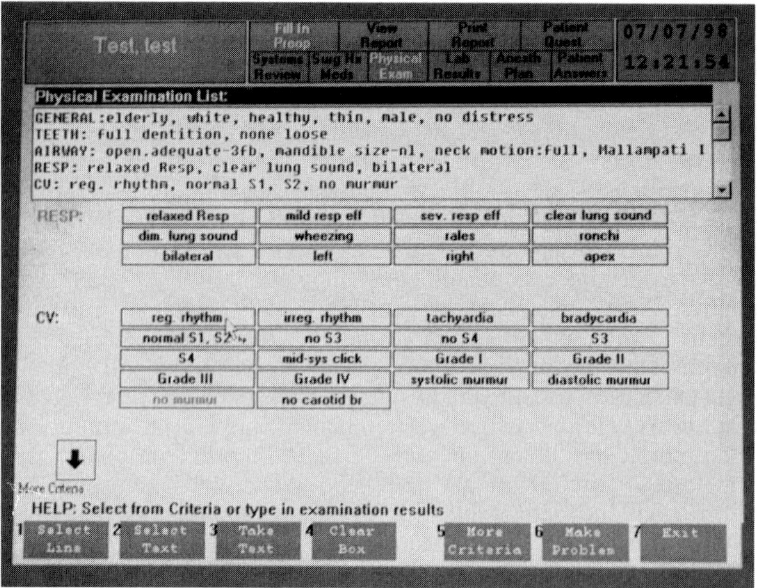


**Figure 6.** Example of physician entry electronic medical records screen which allows canned text to be easily entered with mouse clicks, but which also allows for direct free text typing.

Pre-anaesthetic evaluation systems should be based on a multitasking, graphical computer operating system such as Windows95 and WindowNT or X-Windows. This allows staff and physicians to maintain contact with multiple data sources simultaneously. For example, the physician may research a medical problem using MEDLINE (either via the internet or through a commercial product based on multiple CD-ROMs) while simultaneously reviewing the exact details of a diagnostic test related in the hospital-wide medical records system and simultaneously entering data into a specialized departmental pre-anaesthetic evaluation system (Broering, 1991). Such operating systems normally also make it easy for the physician to copy text electronically from one application to another. This can be extremely beneficial, allowing great reductions in entry time and frustration (Gibby et al 1996a). There are security and confidentiality risks to be considered, however. Medical records information should never be copied and sent to another individual or group without explicit patient permission. The potential damage that could be done by e-mailing patient information is large. There are potential solutions to these problems that can be implemented in the 'cut' or 'copy' routines of specialized computerized medical records systems.

Reliance on an advanced database, usually based on Structured Query Language (SQL) access is favourable. Newer systems will move to 'object databases' which enforce an even higher degree of structure and access control to the data, improving maintainability.

The confidentiality of patient medical records should be carefully considered when evaluating medical records products and for this reason in the United States the JCAHO requires that electronic systems maintain the confidentiality of patient medical records. The essential items that should be considered are as follows (Campbell et al, 1997).

- *User authentication.* An absolute necessity to allow for the possibility of electronic signatures (Noel, 1991). Identity of users may be determined by secure passwords, smart cards or smart buttons (Dallas Semiconductor, Austin, TX; Figure 7) or by biometric techniques such as iris scan, fingerprint, face or palm scan. For non-biometric methods, the users must be required to sign documents promising not to release their password or other identifier to others.
- *Authorization.* Determine whether the user is allowed access to the information, based on permission of patient.
- *Security.* Unauthorized users must not be able to read transmissions; usually prevented by encryption. Systems which pass 'clear text' (unencrypted) over network cables, even if only within the institution, are not secure. Protection of the numerical 'key' must be assured.
- *Reliability.* Data must be protected from erasure; for long-term reliability, CD-ROM back-ups are suggested.
- *Journalling.* All activities of the database should be recorded so that, in the event of database corruption, its contents can be recreated. Databases built to be accessed via SQL often have journalling built in.

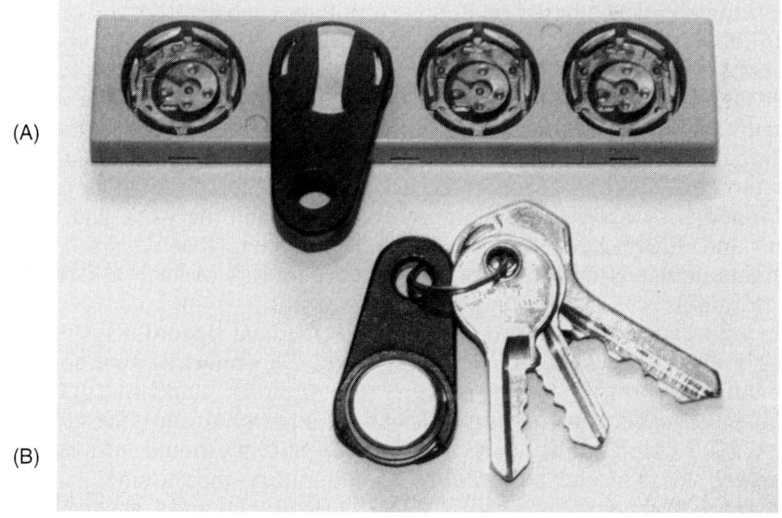


**Figure 7.** (A) Encapsulated smart chip, inside the battery-like 'button' structure to the left. Button is snapped into a receptacle to allow immediate interrogation of its unique identifying number and electronic 'key'. (B) Conventional key on same ring for comparison. Dallas Semiconductor.

- *Audit.* All activities of users should be recorded; a major deterrent to unauthorized actions, but requires intensive effort to review.
- *Non-repudiation.* Activities of users must be provable so that they cannot deny the action; usually accomplished by requiring their transmissions to be encrypted by a key under their sole control.

While identification of the user can be accomplished by passwords, this simple approach is fraught with problems and frustrations for the users, who are tempted to write down complicated passwords (providing a method of possible attack), or to share them or to choose simple words as passwords, allowing attacks by dictionary-based foes. Even if encrypted, simple passwords are insecure because the attacker can often encrypt the entire dictionary and try with each possible choice. A combination with a physical token (such as smart card or hermetically sealed electronic 'button') may be better. Many identification methods have the drawback that they are transitory: passwords, magnetic strips and barcodes prove identity only at the moment of presentation. Further barcodes can be copied; magnetic strips can be erased (see 'denial of service' attack, below) and even copied by astute foes. Smart cards or buttons that cannot be copied or changed, and whose presence is continuously required in a receptacle, when combined with a reasonable password may provide good identification, and represent a solution to many of the problems described.

While most anaesthesia departments will be concerned over the risks of intruders gaining access to confidential patient electronic records, once a system is integrated into their practice, they will become even more concerned about downtime due to system failures. To reduce downtime, networking should be based on a 'star' topology such as 10BaseT or wireless (Gibby et al, 1997b), rather than on the older coaxial 'bus' topology. Network servers should have battery back-up to protect data in the event of power loss, and should properly and gracefully shut down in the event of exhaustion of the battery. A related intruder attack is 'denial of service', in which the intruder will attempt to cause system failures to provoke users to force the administrator to remove password or other protections to give them emergency access. Maintaining a solid reliable network and server system and utilizing a reasonable protection system that does not make inordinate demands on the users will reduce the risk of such a 'denial of service' attack.

For interconnections between different medical records systems, a coding system known as HL7 ('Health Level 7'), (referring to a code for communicating actual test results) is the premier standard, but it is significantly inadequate for transmission of structured anaesthesia information. HL7 compatibility (which is seldom perfect) should, however, be guaranteed to facilitate connections to laboratory measurements. More finely grained standards, such as SNOMED (Rothwell and Cote, 1996) for recording patient evaluations, are unfortunately extremely tedious to use. The future should bring more useful solutions. Efforts to connect between institutions are underway (Grant et al, 1995).

## SUMMARY

The development of the outpatient, at least day-of-surgery admission, model for most surgical procedures in the United States has brought many changes to the pre-anaesthetic evaluation. For the greatest efficiency and throughput, the pre-anaesthetic evaluation clinic is recommended. Such clinics can substantially reduce hospital costs and improve the satisfaction of patients. The field of anaesthesiology is already a leader in the development of direct physician entry electronic medical records; as technology improves, additional institutions will add departmental pre-anaesthetic evaluation systems. Linking these to hospital-wide systems will improve local care. Linking local systems to a nationwide system will allow better nationwide care and may allow for the development of wide-ranging outcome studies of anaesthetic practice.

## REFERENCES


American Society of Anesthesiologists (1987) *Basic Standards for Preanesthetic Care*. Park Ridge, IL: American Society of Anesthesiologists.

American Society of Anesthesiologists (1993) *Statement on Routine Preoperative Laboratory and Diagnostic Screening*. Park Ridge, IL: American Society of Anesthesiologists.

American Society of Anesthesiologists (1996) *Managed Care Contracting: Considerations for Anesthesiologists*, p 15. Park Ridge, IL: Squire Sanders & Dempsey, American Society of Anesthesiologists.

Auxter S (1998). Implementing the new HCFA/AMA panels: is your hospital ready for the switch? *Clinical Laboratory News* (*http://www.aacc.org/cln/*198features/Jan98hcfafeat.html).

Bergeron BP (1996) Voice recognition: an enabling technology for modern health care? *Proceedings of the American Medical Informatics Association, Annual Fall Symposium Supplement* pp 802–806.

Broering C (1991) The MAClinical workstation project at Georgetown University. *Bulletin of the Medical Library Association* **79:** 276–281.

*Campbell SG, Gibby GL & Collingwood S (1997) The internet and electronic transmission of medical records. *Journal of Clinical Monitoring* **13:** 325–334.

Dambro M, Weiss BD, McClure CL & Vutoro AF (1988) An unsuccessful experience with computerized medical records in an academic medical center. *Journal of Medical Education* **63:** 617–623.

Davies JM, Pagenkopf D, Todd K et al (1994) Comparison of selection of preoperative laboratory tests: the computer vs. the anaesthetist. *Canadian Journal of Anaesthesia* **41:** 1156–1160.

East TD (1992) Computers in the ICU: panacea or plague? *Respiratory Care* **37:** 170–180.

Edsall DW (1991) Quality assessment with a computerized anesthesia information management system (AIMS). *Quality Review Bulletin* **17:** 182–193.

Elsass P (1990) The psychological effect of three different forms of patient information. Clinical Psychological Department, Psychiatric Hospital, Risskov. *Danish Medical Bulletin* **37:** 185–188.

Federal Register (1996) *Medicare Program; Revisions to Payment Policies and Five-Year Review of and Adjustments to the Relative Value Units Under the Physician Fee Schedule for Calendar Year 1997, Final Rule; Physician Fee Schedule Update for Calendar Year 1997 and Physician Volume Performance Standard Rates of Increase for Federal Fiscal Year 1997, Notice. Federal Register* 61 (227), Rules and Regulations, section IV.B.3, 'Anesthesia', pp 59530–59531.

*Fischer SP (1996) Development and effectiveness of an anesthesia preoperative evaluation clinic in a teaching hospital. *Anesthesiology* **85:** 196–206.

*Gibby GL (1997) Anesthesia information-management systems: their role in risk-versus cost-assessment and outcomes research. *Journal of Cardiothoracic and Vascular Anesthesia* **11 (supplement 1):** 2–5.

Gibby GL & Schwab WK (1998) Availability of records in an outpatient preanesthetic evaluation clinic. *Journal of Clinical Monitoring and Computing* **14:** 385–391.

Gibby GL, Lemeer G & Jackson K (1996a) Use of data from a hospital online medical records system by physicians during preanesthetic evaluation. *Journal of Clinical Monitoring* **12:** 405–408.

Gibby GL, Schwab WK & Goede R (1996b) Availability of medical records to the outpatient preanesthetic clinic. *International Journal of Clinical Monitoring and Computation* **13:** 198–199 (abstract).

*Gibby GL, Schwab WK, Jackson K et al (1996c) A computerized preanesthetic evaluation medical records system: development, use, and administrative impact. *Surgery Services Management* **2:** 29–35.

*Gibby GL, Paulus DA, Sirota DJ et al (1997a) Computerized pre-anesthetic evaluation results in additional abstracted comorbidity diagnoses. *Journal of Clinical Monitoring* **13:** 35–41.

Gibby GL, Schwab WK & Miller WC (1997b) Evaluation of electrosurgical interference to low-power spread-spectrum local area net transceivers. *Journal of Clinical Monitoring* **13:** 345–348.

Grajek SE, Calarco P, Frawley SJ et al (1997) Evaluating IAIMS at Yale: information access. *Journal of the American Medical Informatics Association* **4:** 138–149.

Grant A, Delisle E, Dubois S et al (1995) Implementation of a province-wide computerized network in Quebec: the Famus Project. *MD Computing* **12:** 45–49.

Hsia DC, Ahern CA, Ritchie BP et al (1992) Medicare reimbursement accuracy under the prospective payment system, 1985 to 1988. *Journal of the American Medical Association* **268:** 896–899.

Jackson KI, Gibby GL, Arroyo AA & Principle JC (1993) Preliminary evaluation of an artificial neural network for predicting patient outcome in anesthesia. *Anesthesia and Analgesia* **76:** S158 (abstract).

*Jackson KI, Gibby GL & van der Aa JJ (1994) The efficiency of preoperative evaluation: a comparison of computerized and paper recording systems. *Journal of Clinical Monitoring* **10:** 189–193.

Lack JA, Stuart-Taylor M & Tecklenburg A (1994) An anaesthetic minimum dataset and report format. *British Journal of Anaesthesia* **73:** 256–260.

Louagie Y, Buche M, Jamart J et al (1995) Operative risk assessment in coronary artery bypass surgery, 1990–1993: evaluation of perioperative variables. *Thoracic and Cardiovascular Surgery* **43(3):** 134–141.

Lutner RE, Roizen MF, Stocking CB et al (1991) The automated interview versus the personal interview: do patient responses to preoperative health questions differ? *Anesthesiology* **75:** 394–400.

Mark L, Schauber J, Gibby G, Drake JL (1996) Effective dissemination of critical airway information: the Medic Alert National Difficult Airway/Intubation Registry. In Benumof JL (ed.) *Airway Management: Principles and Practice*, pp 931–943.

McDonald CJ & Tierney WM (1988) Computer-stored medical records: their future role in medical practice. *Journal of the American Medical Association* **259:** 3433–3440.

Murphy SN & Barnett GO (1996) Achieving automated narrative text interpretation using phrases in the electronic medical record. *Proceedings of the American Medical Informatics Association, Annual Fall Symposium Supplement*, pp 532–536.

*Noel LA (1991) Electronic signatures: a brief overview. *Journal of AMRA* **62:** 38–41.

O'Dell DV, Tape TG & Compbell JR (1991) Increasing physician acceptance and use of the computerized ambulatory medical record. *Proceedings of the Annual Symposium on Computer Applications in Medical Care*, pp 848–852.

O'Rourke MR & Smith R (1975) A practical system of computerized medical records for documentation and decision making in the coronary care ward. *Medical Journal of Australia* **1:** 301–304.

Painter PC (1997) The laboratory, physicians, and medical necessity: making sure your lab is in compliance. *Clinical Laboratory News* (http://www.aacc.org/cln/97features/sep97feat.html).

*Roizen MF (1994) Cost-effective preoperative laboratory testing. *Journal of the American Medical Association*. **271:** 319–320.

Rothwell DJ & Cote RA (1996) Managing information with SNOMED: understanding the model. *Proceedings of the American Medical Informatics Association. Annual Fall Symposium Supplement*, pp 80–83.

Safran C, Rury C, Rind DM & Taylor WC (1991) A computer-based outpatient medical record for a teaching hospital. *Clinical Computing* **8:** 291–299.

Schwab WK, Jackson KI, Layon AJ et al (1996) Graphical patient tracking system. *Journal of Clinical Monitoring* **12:** 48 (abstract).

Smith NT, Brient RA, Pettus DC et al (1990) Recognition accuracy with a voice-recognition system designed for anesthesia record keeping. *Journal of Clinical Monitoring* **6:** 299–306.

Society for Technology in Anesthesia (1998) Electronic availability of anesthesia records, *http://gasnet.med.yale.edu/sta/edatamgt/PolicyStatement.htm.*

Stead WW & Hammond WE (1983) Computerized medical records: a new resource for clinical decision making. *Journal of Medical Systems* **7:** 213–220.

Stead WW, Hammond WE & Straube MJ (1983) A chartless record—is it adequate? *Journal of Medical Systems* **7:** 103–109.

Thompson DC, Benner SA & Witt C (1995) Integrating clinical research data with a clinical data repository. *HIMSS Proceedings*, vol. 1, pp 271–281. Healthcare Information and Management Systems Society.

Tierney WM, Miller ME, Overhage JM & McDonald CJ (1993) Physician inpatient order writing on microcomputer workstations: effects on resource utilization. *Journal of the American Medical Association* **269:** 379–383.

*Tompkins BM, Tompkins WJ, Loder E & Noonan AF (1980) A computer-assisted preanesthesia interview: value of a computer-generated summary of patient's historical information in the pre-anesthetic visit. *Anesthesia and Analgesia* **59:** 3–10.

Wyatt JC (1994) Clinical data systems, part 1: data and medical records. *Lancet* **344:** 1543–1547.

# Index

Note: Page numbers of article titles are in **bold** type.